JUICING FOR HEALING

Tailored Juice Plans for Managing Rheumatoid Arthritis, Type 2 Diabetes, IBS, Eczema, Hashimoto's Thyroiditis, and more.

Theresa Walsh

Table of Contents

Introduction

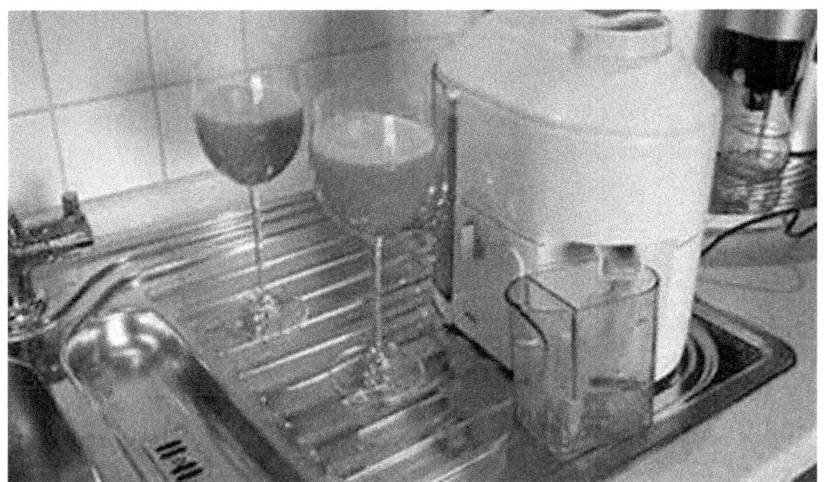

The Power of Juicing for Holistic Healing

Juicing stands as a powerful and transformative practice, not merely as a refreshing beverage option but as a holistic approach to healing the body, mind, and spirit. At its core, juicing harnesses the inherent therapeutic properties of fresh fruits and vegetables to promote overall well-being, offering a myriad of benefits that extend beyond mere hydration. Understanding the depth of this practice unveils the profound impact it can have on one's journey towards holistic healing.

At the heart of juicing lies the concentration of vital nutrients, including vitamins, minerals, antioxidants, and enzymes, derived from an array of colorful and nutrient-dense plant-based ingredients. This concentrated elixir provides the body with a potent dose of bioavailable nutrients, enhancing its ability to repair, regenerate, and defend against external stressors. The richness of these nutrients not only fuels the physical body but also plays a crucial role in supporting mental clarity and emotional balance.

One of the fundamental aspects of juicing for holistic healing is its ability to boost the immune system. The synergistic combination of vitamins like C and E, along with antioxidants such as beta-carotene and flavonoids, fortifies the body's defense mechanisms. Regular consumption of immune-boosting juices contributes to resilience against infections, viruses, and other ailments, fostering a foundation of health from within.

Beyond physical health, the practice of juicing extends its healing touch to mental and emotional well-being. The vibrant colors and flavors of fresh juices invigorate the senses, creating a sensory experience that transcends the act of consumption. This sensory stimulation can uplift mood, reduce stress, and contribute to an overall sense of vitality. The link between nutrition and mental health is increasingly recognized, and juicing becomes a tangible means of supporting emotional balance through nourishing the body with essential nutrients.

Juicing also serves as a catalyst for detoxification, aiding the body in eliminating accumulated toxins and promoting cellular regeneration. The hydrating and cleansing properties of fresh juices support the liver, kidneys, and other organs involved in the body's natural detox processes. As toxins are expelled, the body's energy is redirected towards healing and restoration, fostering a renewed sense of vitality.

Holistic healing encompasses the integration of the body, mind, and spirit, and juicing becomes a conduit for aligning these interconnected elements. The ritual of preparing and consuming fresh juices becomes an intentional act, fostering mindfulness and presence. This mindful approach extends beyond the physical act of juicing, seeping into other aspects of life and promoting a more conscious and balanced lifestyle.

In the realm of holistic healing, juicing can also be seen as a form of self-care and self-love. It provides individuals with the opportunity to prioritize their well-being, nurturing themselves from the inside out. The act of selecting, preparing, and savoring fresh ingredients becomes a mindful expression of self-love, fostering a positive relationship with one's body and overall health.

In essence, the power of juicing for holistic healing lies not only in the nutrient-packed elixirs it produces but in the transformative journey it initiates. It encourages individuals to reevaluate their relationship with food, embrace intentional living, and embark on a path of holistic well-being that encompasses the body, mind, and spirit. As the vibrant hues of fresh juices infuse life into each sip, they become a testament to the potential for healing that resides within the simple act of nourishing oneself with the gifts of nature.

Understanding the Impact of Nutrition on Chronic Conditions

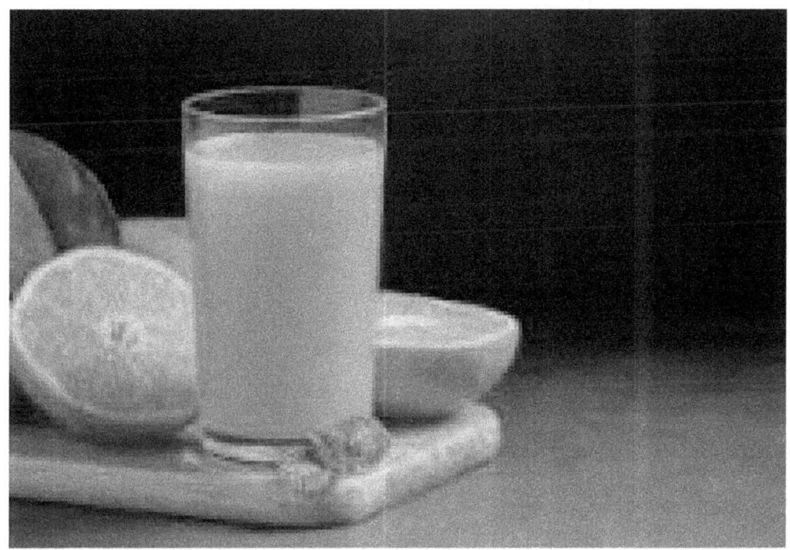

The link between nutrition and chronic conditions is a profound and intricate aspect of overall health. Recognizing the impact that dietary choices have on chronic ailments is essential for those seeking not only symptom management but true healing from within. This exploration delves into the nuanced relationship between nutrition and chronic conditions, emphasizing the transformative potential of nutrient-rich choices in fostering well-being.

At the core of understanding this relationship is the acknowledgment that food serves as more than mere sustenance; it is a powerful tool that can either exacerbate or alleviate chronic conditions. For individuals grappling with ailments such as rheumatoid arthritis, multiple sclerosis, type 2 diabetes, and other chronic health challenges, the role of nutrition extends beyond calorie intake to influencing inflammation, immune function, and overall bodily processes.

Certain nutrients possess anti-inflammatory properties that can be particularly beneficial for managing chronic inflammatory conditions. Omega-3 fatty acids found in fatty fish, flaxseeds, and walnuts, for example, have been associated with reduced inflammation and improved joint health, making them valuable components of a diet aimed at managing conditions like rheumatoid arthritis.

Balancing blood sugar levels is paramount for individuals dealing with type 2 diabetes. Understanding the glycemic index of foods and incorporating complex carbohydrates, fiber-rich vegetables, and lean proteins can contribute to stable blood sugar levels, aiding in diabetes management. The intricate dance between nutrients, insulin response, and energy metabolism plays a pivotal role in the nutritional approach to this chronic condition.

Moreover, the impact of nutrition on gut health is gaining increasing recognition in the context of chronic conditions. For individuals with inflammatory bowel diseases (IBD) or autoimmune disorders like Hashimoto's thyroiditis, maintaining a healthy gut microbiome is crucial. Incorporating probiotic-rich foods, fiber, and fermented options can support gut health and contribute to the management of these conditions.

Understanding the role of specific nutrients, vitamins, and minerals in chronic conditions becomes a key element in crafting a healing-oriented diet. Antioxidants found in fruits and vegetables, such as vitamin C and E, play a crucial role in neutralizing free radicals and reducing oxidative stress, contributing to the overall well-being of individuals managing chronic health challenges.

Beyond individual nutrients, the overall composition of one's diet, including the balance of macronutrients (carbohydrates, proteins, and fats), plays a pivotal role in managing chronic conditions. Adopting an anti-inflammatory diet, characterized by whole foods, lean proteins, and healthy fats, can be instrumental in mitigating the impact of inflammation associated with various chronic ailments.

The personalized nature of nutritional impact on chronic conditions emphasizes the need for tailored dietary plans. Each chronic condition may require a nuanced approach, and working with healthcare professionals, nutritionists, or dietitians becomes crucial in designing a plan that aligns with individual health goals and addresses specific challenges.

In conclusion, understanding the impact of nutrition on chronic conditions is a dynamic and evolving field. It requires a holistic perspective that considers the interconnectedness of nutrients, bodily processes, and the unique needs of individuals dealing with chronic health challenges. By embracing the transformative potential of nutrient-rich choices and adopting a personalized approach to dietary management, individuals can pave the way for healing, resilience, and improved quality of life in the face of chronic conditions.

Chapter 1: The Science Behind Juicing and Healing

The science behind juicing and its healing properties delves into the intricate world of biochemistry and nutrition, unveiling the remarkable transformations that occur when fresh fruits and vegetables are converted into vibrant elixirs. At the core of this science is the profound impact of bioactive compounds, vitamins, and minerals on the body's physiological processes, setting the stage for holistic healing.

Freshly pressed juices offer a concentrated source of essential nutrients, including vitamins A, C, and E, as well as an array of powerful antioxidants. These bioactive compounds play pivotal roles in neutralizing free radicals, reducing inflammation, and supporting cellular repair and regeneration. The synergy of these nutrients creates a nutritional powerhouse that can contribute to the prevention and management of various health conditions.

Enzymes, another crucial component found in fresh juices, aid in the digestion and absorption of nutrients. These living compounds facilitate the breakdown of food into its essential components, ensuring optimal nutrient assimilation. The preservation of enzymes in raw, freshly juiced fruits and vegetables enhances the bioavailability of nutrients, promoting a more efficient utilization of these vital elements by the body.

The low processing temperatures involved in juicing help maintain the integrity of heat-sensitive nutrients. This preservation of nutritional content distinguishes juicing from other forms of food processing that may compromise the potency of vitamins and enzymes. The resulting juice becomes a bioavailable elixir, delivering a concentrated burst of health-promoting compounds directly to the cells.

Moreover, the hydration provided by fresh juices supports cellular function and enhances overall bodily functions. Proper hydration is foundational to health, and the liquid form of juices contributes to maintaining optimal fluid balance. This hydrating effect also extends to the skin, promoting a radiant complexion and supporting the body's natural detoxification processes.

In essence, the science behind juicing and healing unveils the nutritional alchemy that occurs when fresh produce is transformed into liquid vitality. It is a symphony of vitamins, antioxidants, enzymes, and hydration that collaborates to promote well-being at the cellular level. Understanding this scientific foundation empowers individuals to harness the healing potential of juicing, making it a potent and delicious tool in the pursuit of optimal health.

Nutritional Foundations for Disease Management

Nutritional foundations for disease management serve as the cornerstone of a proactive and holistic approach to health. Recognizing the profound impact of dietary choices on various health conditions lays the groundwork for promoting well-being, managing symptoms, and supporting the body's natural healing processes. This exploration delves into the essential nutritional elements that form the foundation for effective disease management.

1. Macro and Micronutrient Balance: A balanced intake of macronutrients (carbohydrates, proteins, and fats) and micronutrients (vitamins and minerals) is crucial for disease management. Tailoring the proportions of these nutrients to individual health conditions helps optimize energy levels, support bodily functions, and address specific nutritional needs associated with various illnesses.

2. Antioxidant-Rich Foods: Antioxidants play a pivotal role in neutralizing free radicals, which contribute to inflammation and cellular damage. Incorporating a variety of colorful fruits and vegetables rich in antioxidants, such as vitamin C, E, and beta-carotene, helps mitigate oxidative stress and supports overall health.

3. Omega-3 Fatty Acids: For conditions involving inflammation, such as rheumatoid arthritis and autoimmune disorders, incorporating omega-3 fatty acids is beneficial. Found in fatty fish, flaxseeds, and walnuts, these essential fatty acids have anti-inflammatory properties that can contribute to symptom management and improved joint health.

4. Fiber for Gut Health: Fiber plays a crucial role in supporting gut health and managing conditions like irritable bowel syndrome (IBS) or inflammatory bowel diseases. A diet rich in soluble and insoluble fiber from whole grains, fruits, and vegetables promotes regular bowel movements, aids digestion, and fosters a healthy gut microbiome.

5. Blood Sugar Management: For individuals dealing with type 2 diabetes, maintaining stable blood sugar levels is paramount. Choosing complex carbohydrates, high-fiber foods, and incorporating lean proteins helps regulate blood sugar, supporting overall glycemic control.

6. Adequate Hydration: Proper hydration is fundamental for all aspects of health and is particularly important in disease management. Staying well-hydrated supports cellular function, aids in detoxification processes, and contributes to overall bodily well-being.

7. Individualized Nutrition Plans: Recognizing the unique nutritional needs of individuals with specific health conditions underscores the importance of personalized nutrition plans. Working with healthcare professionals or registered dietitians ensures that dietary recommendations align with individual health goals and medical considerations.

8. Mindful Eating Practices: Beyond specific nutrients, adopting mindful eating practices contributes to disease management. Being attentive to hunger and fullness cues, practicing portion control, and savoring each bite fosters a positive relationship with food and supports overall well-being.

In essence, nutritional foundations for disease management extend beyond mere sustenance; they represent a strategic and intentional approach to leveraging the healing power of food. By understanding and incorporating these foundational principles into daily dietary choices, individuals can proactively contribute to their health, fostering resilience, and enhancing their quality of life in the face of various health conditions.

How Juicing Supports the Body's Natural Healing Processes

Juicing stands as a vibrant gateway to harnessing the body's innate ability to heal and rejuvenate. Beyond its refreshing and flavorful appeal, the process of juicing offers a concentrated infusion of essential nutrients, antioxidants, and enzymes, empowering the body's natural healing processes in a profound and dynamic manner.

1. Nutrient Density and Bioavailability: Freshly pressed juices are a treasure trove of vitamins, minerals, and phytonutrients derived from an assortment of fruits and vegetables. The process of juicing extracts these nutrients in liquid form, significantly enhancing their concentration. This nutrient density ensures that the body receives an abundant supply of essential elements, promoting optimal cellular function and metabolic processes. The liquid nature of juices also enhances bioavailability, facilitating easier absorption of these vital nutrients into the bloodstream.

2. Cellular Repair and Regeneration: The powerful antioxidants present in freshly juiced fruits and vegetables play a pivotal role in combating oxidative stress and free radicals within the body. This antioxidant defense bolsters the body's ability to repair damaged cells and tissues, supporting overall cellular health. Regular consumption of antioxidant-rich juices contributes to a protective environment that aids in the prevention of chronic diseases and promotes longevity.

3. Enzymatic Support for Digestion: Enzymes are living compounds crucial for the breakdown and absorption of nutrients. Raw, freshly juiced fruits and vegetables contain naturally occurring enzymes that facilitate the digestion and assimilation of essential nutrients. This enzymatic support ensures that the body can efficiently extract the maximum nutritional value from the juices, fostering a robust digestive system and enhancing nutrient utilization.

4. Hydration and Detoxification: Proper hydration is fundamental to the body's detoxification processes. Juicing, with its high-water content, contributes to hydration at the cellular level. Adequate hydration supports the flushing out of toxins, promoting kidney function and enhancing overall detoxification. The hydrating effect of juices also contributes to skin health, giving it a radiant and rejuvenated appearance.

5. Anti-Inflammatory Properties: Chronic inflammation is at the root of many health issues. The anti-inflammatory compounds present in fresh juices, such as polyphenols and flavonoids, contribute to reducing inflammation within the body. This anti-inflammatory support is particularly beneficial for conditions like arthritis and autoimmune disorders, where inflammation plays a significant role in symptomatology.

6. Immune System Boost: The abundance of vitamins, especially vitamin C, in freshly pressed juices enhances the body's immune response. These immune-boosting nutrients fortify the body's defense mechanisms, providing resilience against infections and illnesses. Regular consumption of immune-supportive juices becomes a proactive measure in maintaining overall health and well-being.

7. Cellular Hygiene and Waste Elimination: Juicing supports the body's natural processes of cellular hygiene and waste elimination. The influx of nutrients facilitates cellular repair, while the liquid nature of juices aids in the removal of metabolic waste products. This dual action contributes to maintaining cellular health and promoting an environment conducive to the body's intrinsic healing capabilities.

In essence, how juicing supports the body's natural healing processes lies in the intricate dance of nutrients, antioxidants, and enzymes present in freshly pressed juices. It becomes a transformative elixir that nourishes, revitalizes, and aligns with the body's inherent capacity to heal. Embracing juicing as a part of a balanced and health-conscious lifestyle becomes a proactive choice in fostering holistic well-being and embracing the vitality that nature's bounty can offer.

Chapter 2: Choosing the Right Ingredients for Specific Conditions

Building a Foundation: Essential Nutrients for Overall Health

Creating a robust foundation for overall health hinges on the conscious intake of a diverse array of essential nutrients. These fundamental elements, derived from a balanced and nutrient-rich diet, play a pivotal role in supporting bodily functions, promoting vitality, and preventing the onset of various health issues. Delving into the intricacies of these essential nutrients unveils their unique contributions to building a foundation for optimal well-being.

1. Proteins: Proteins are the building blocks of life, serving as crucial components for the structure, function, and regulation of tissues and organs. Essential amino acids, obtained through protein-rich foods like lean meats, dairy, beans, and nuts, play a vital role in cellular repair, immune function, and the synthesis of enzymes and hormones.

2. Carbohydrates: Carbohydrates serve as the primary source of energy for the body. Complex carbohydrates, found in whole grains, fruits, and vegetables, provide sustained energy and essential fiber for digestive health. Balancing carbohydrate intake is essential for maintaining stable blood sugar levels and preventing energy fluctuations.

3. Fats: Healthy fats, including omega-3 and omega-6 fatty acids, are essential for brain health, hormone production, and the absorption of fat-soluble vitamins (A, D, E, K). Sources of healthy fats include fatty fish, avocados, nuts, and olive oil. Striking a balance between different types of fats contributes to cardiovascular health and overall well-being.

4. Vitamins: Vitamins are micronutrients vital for various physiological processes. Vitamin C supports immune function, collagen synthesis, and antioxidant activity. B-vitamins, including B12 and folate, play roles in energy metabolism and DNA synthesis. Obtaining a spectrum of vitamins from fruits, vegetables, whole grains, and lean proteins ensures a comprehensive nutritional profile.

5. Minerals: Minerals, such as calcium, magnesium, potassium, and iron, are essential for bone health, muscle function, and overall metabolic balance. Dairy products, leafy greens, nuts, and lean meats are rich sources of these vital minerals. Maintaining proper mineral balance contributes to optimal cellular function.

6. Fiber: Dietary fiber is indispensable for digestive health and the prevention of constipation. It also helps regulate blood sugar levels and supports heart health. Whole grains, fruits, vegetables, and legumes are excellent sources of dietary fiber. A fiber-rich diet contributes to overall gut health and assists in weight management.

7. Water: Hydration is foundational to overall health. Water plays a crucial role in nutrient transport, temperature regulation, and waste elimination. Adequate hydration supports cognitive function, skin health, and the efficient functioning of bodily systems. Drinking an ample amount of water daily is a cornerstone of maintaining optimal health.

8. Antioxidants: Antioxidants, such as vitamins C and E, beta-carotene, and selenium, combat oxidative stress and neutralize free radicals in the body. These compounds, found in colorful fruits and vegetables, contribute to cellular protection, immune support, and the prevention of chronic diseases.

Building a foundation for overall health involves the harmonious integration of these essential nutrients into daily dietary choices. A diverse and well-rounded diet, rich in whole foods, ensures that the body receives the necessary elements for optimal function, resilience, and longevity. Embracing nutritional balance becomes a proactive step towards not just treating ailments but cultivating a lifestyle that fosters enduring health and well-being.

Tailoring Juicing Ingredients for Rheumatoid Arthritis

Rheumatoid Arthritis (RA), characterized by chronic inflammation of the joints, demands a thoughtful and holistic approach to managing symptoms and promoting overall well-being. Juicing, with its potent array of anti-inflammatory and nutrient-rich ingredients, emerges as a valuable adjunct in the management of RA. Tailoring juicing ingredients for individuals with RA involves a meticulous selection of fruits, vegetables, and herbs known for their anti-inflammatory properties and their ability to provide essential nutrients that support joint health.

1. Pineapple and Turmeric Elixir: Pineapple, rich in bromelain, and turmeric, containing curcumin, team up to create a powerful anti-inflammatory elixir. Bromelain exhibits anti-inflammatory and analgesic properties, potentially assisting in reducing joint pain and swelling. Curcumin, a potent compound in turmeric, is renowned for its anti-inflammatory and antioxidant effects. Combining these ingredients in a juicing concoction provides a refreshing and therapeutic beverage that may contribute to easing the symptoms of RA.

2. Leafy Greens for Nutrient Density: Dark leafy greens, such as kale, spinach, and Swiss chard, bring a wealth of nutrients to the table. Rich in vitamins, minerals, and antioxidants, these greens offer essential nutrients like vitamin K, which supports bone health, and antioxidants that combat oxidative stress associated with RA. The inclusion of leafy greens in juicing ensures a nutrient-dense elixir that nourishes the body at the cellular level, potentially aiding in the overall management of RA symptoms.

3. Ginger and Citrus Infusion: Ginger, celebrated for its anti-inflammatory and analgesic properties, pairs seamlessly with citrus fruits like oranges and lemons. Gingerol, the active compound in ginger, exhibits anti-inflammatory effects that may be beneficial for individuals with RA. Citrus fruits, high in vitamin C and flavonoids, contribute to immune support and collagen synthesis, potentially supporting joint health. This zesty and invigorating juice infusion not only tantalizes the taste buds but also provides a refreshing way to incorporate anti-inflammatory elements into the diet.

4. Berry Blast for Antioxidant Power: Berries, such as blueberries, strawberries, and raspberries, boast a vibrant array of antioxidants, including anthocyanins and quercetin. These antioxidants contribute to reducing inflammation and oxidative stress, common factors in RA. Incorporating a berry blast into the juicing repertoire not only satisfies sweet cravings but also harnesses the potential of these colorful gems to support joint health and overall well-being.

5. Celery and Cucumber Cooler: Celery and cucumber, with their high-water content and anti-inflammatory properties, form a hydrating and soothing juice blend. Celery contains compounds like apigenin, which exhibits anti-inflammatory effects, while cucumbers contribute hydration and additional anti-inflammatory compounds. This cooling combination not only supports overall hydration, crucial for joint health, but also provides a gentle and refreshing addition to the anti-inflammatory juicing arsenal.

6. Omega-3 Rich Flaxseed Elixir: Flaxseeds, abundant in omega-3 fatty acids, particularly alpha-linolenic acid (ALA), offer anti-inflammatory benefits that may be beneficial for individuals with RA. Omega-3 fatty acids are known for their potential to reduce inflammation and may contribute to joint health. Including ground flaxseeds in a juicing concoction brings a nutty flavor and a nutritional punch, enhancing the omega-3 profile of the beverage.

Tailoring juicing ingredients for Rheumatoid Arthritis involves a thoughtful combination of these anti-inflammatory and nutrient-dense elements. While juicing alone is not a cure for RA, incorporating these vibrant and healing ingredients into the diet may complement traditional treatments, offering a holistic approach to managing inflammation and supporting overall joint health. As with any dietary changes, consulting with healthcare professionals or nutritionists ensures that juicing plans align with individual health goals and medical considerations, enhancing the potential benefits for individuals navigating the challenges of Rheumatoid Arthritis.

Managing Multiple Sclerosis through Targeted Nutrition

Multiple Sclerosis (MS), a chronic autoimmune disease affecting the central nervous system, prompts individuals to explore comprehensive approaches to manage symptoms and promote overall health. Targeted nutrition plays a crucial role in this endeavor, offering a means to support the body's resilience, minimize inflammation, and foster overall well-being in the face of MS.

1. Omega-3 Fatty Acids: Incorporating omega-3 fatty acids into the diet is particularly beneficial for individuals with MS. Fatty fish, flaxseeds, chia seeds, and walnuts are rich sources of these essential fats. Omega-3s exhibit anti-inflammatory properties, potentially aiding in reducing inflammation associated with MS and supporting overall neurological health.

2. Vitamin D: Vitamin D is vital for individuals with MS, as it plays a role in immune function and may contribute to symptom management. Exposure to sunlight and vitamin D-rich foods such as fatty fish, fortified dairy products, and mushrooms can help maintain optimal vitamin D levels.

3. Antioxidant-Rich Foods: Berries, dark leafy greens, and colorful fruits and vegetables provide a plethora of antioxidants. These compounds combat oxidative stress and free radicals, contributing to overall cellular health. Including antioxidant-rich foods in the diet may potentially help manage oxidative damage associated with MS.

4. Gut-Healthy Foods: Maintaining gut health is increasingly recognized as a crucial aspect of managing autoimmune conditions. Probiotics from sources like yogurt, kefir, and fermented foods promote a healthy gut microbiome, potentially influencing immune function and inflammation.

5. Whole Grains and Fiber: Whole grains and fiber-rich foods such as oats, brown rice, legumes, and vegetables support digestive health and contribute to a stable blood sugar level. This can be particularly relevant for individuals with MS, as fluctuations in blood sugar levels may impact energy levels and overall well-being.

6. Adequate Hydration: Staying well-hydrated is essential for individuals with MS. Proper hydration supports overall bodily functions, including cognitive function and temperature regulation. Water, herbal teas, and hydrating foods like watermelon contribute to maintaining optimal hydration.

7. Low-Fat, Balanced Diet: Adopting a low-fat and balanced diet can be beneficial for individuals with MS. Lean proteins, healthy fats, and a variety of fruits and vegetables provide essential nutrients without contributing to excessive inflammation.

8. Individualized Nutrition Plans: Recognizing the unique needs of individuals with MS, creating individualized nutrition plans with the guidance of healthcare professionals or registered dietitians is crucial. These professionals can tailor dietary recommendations to address specific symptoms, dietary restrictions, and overall health goals.

While targeted nutrition can be a supportive component in managing Multiple Sclerosis, it is essential to integrate these dietary changes into a comprehensive healthcare plan that includes medical treatment, exercise, and other lifestyle considerations. Consultation with healthcare professionals ensures that nutrition plans align with individual health needs and contribute to a holistic approach to managing MS and fostering overall well-being.

Type 2 Diabetes: Balancing Blood Sugar with Juicing

Type 2 diabetes is a condition characterized by insulin resistance, leading to elevated blood sugar levels. While it's crucial for individuals with diabetes to manage their carbohydrate intake, incorporating fresh juices with the right ingredients can be a flavorful and nutrient-packed approach to help balance blood sugar levels. Juicing can offer a convenient and delicious way to include essential nutrients that support overall health while considering the specific needs of individuals managing diabetes.

1. Selecting Low-Glycemic Fruits and Vegetables: Choosing fruits and vegetables with a low glycemic index is a key consideration for individuals with type 2 diabetes. Low-glycemic foods have a smaller impact on blood sugar levels. Examples include leafy greens, cucumbers, berries, and citrus fruits. Incorporating these ingredients into your juices helps minimize the risk of blood sugar spikes.

2. Fiber-Rich Additions for Sustained Energy: Fiber plays a crucial role in slowing down the absorption of sugar, providing sustained energy and helping to stabilize blood sugar levels. Including high-fiber vegetables like kale, spinach, and broccoli in your juices adds a nutritional boost while contributing to better blood sugar control.

3. Incorporating Lean Proteins: While juices are primarily composed of fruits and vegetables, adding a source of lean protein can enhance the overall nutritional profile and aid in managing blood sugar levels. Ingredients such as Greek yogurt or plant-based protein powders can be blended into your juices for a protein boost without significantly impacting blood sugar.

4. Cinnamon Infusions for Flavor and Potential Benefits:
Cinnamon is not only a flavorful addition to juices but may
also offer potential benefits for individuals with type 2
diabetes. Studies suggest that cinnamon may improve
insulin sensitivity and contribute to better blood sugar
control. Adding a pinch of cinnamon to your juice blends can
enhance both taste and nutritional value.

5. Hydration with Infused Water: Staying well-hydrated
is essential for individuals with diabetes. Infusing water with
slices of citrus fruits, cucumber, and mint can add refreshing
flavor without the added sugars found in many commercial
beverages. Proper hydration supports overall health and can
contribute to better blood sugar management.

6. Portion Control and Monitoring Carbohydrates:
While juicing can be a valuable addition to a diabetes-
friendly diet, it's crucial to practice portion control and
monitor carbohydrate intake. Understanding the
carbohydrate content of your juice recipes and adjusting
portion sizes to fit your individual dietary needs is essential
for maintaining stable blood sugar levels.

**7. Personalized Juicing Plans with Healthcare
Professionals:** Creating personalized juicing plans should
be done in consultation with healthcare professionals or
registered dietitians, especially for individuals with type 2
diabetes. Healthcare providers can provide guidance on
individualized nutritional needs, ensuring that juicing aligns
with diabetes management goals and overall health.

In conclusion, juicing can be a flavorful and nutrient-packed
tool for individuals with type 2 diabetes to include essential
vitamins, minerals, and antioxidants in their diet. The key
lies in choosing the right ingredients, focusing on low-

glycemic options, incorporating fiber, and practicing portion control. By adopting a mindful and personalized approach to juicing, individuals with diabetes can enjoy the benefits of these nutrient-rich beverages while supporting their overall health and blood sugar management.

Here are some of the pros and cons of juicing for people with type 2 diabetes:

Pros

- Juicing can help you increase your intake of fruits and vegetables, which are rich in vitamins, minerals, and phytochemicals that can lower inflammation, prevent disease, and promote overall health.

- Juicing can provide some prebiotics, which are types of carbohydrates that feed the beneficial bacteria in your gut and support digestive health.

- Juicing can help you hydrate, as fruits and vegetables have high water content. Staying hydrated can help regulate blood sugar levels and prevent dehydration, which can worsen diabetes complications.

Cons

- Juicing can raise your blood sugar levels very quickly, as it removes most of the fiber from fruits and vegetables, which slows down the digestion and absorption of carbohydrates. This can lead to spikes and crashes in blood sugar, which can affect your mood, energy, and appetite.

- Juicing can reduce your intake of protein and healthy fats, which are essential for balancing blood sugar, building muscle, and maintaining a healthy weight. Protein and fat also help you feel full and satisfied, which can prevent overeating and cravings.

- Juicing can be expensive, as it requires a lot of fruits and vegetables to make a small amount of juice. It can also be time-consuming and messy, as you need to wash, chop, and juice the produce, and clean the juicer afterwards.

Recommendations

If you have type 2 diabetes and want to try juicing, here are some tips to make it safer and healthier for you:

- Choose low-sugar fruits and vegetables, such as berries, apples, celery, cucumber, kale, spinach, and broccoli. Avoid high-sugar fruits and vegetables, such as grapes, bananas, pineapples, carrots, and beets.

- Add some protein and healthy fat to your juice, such as nuts, seeds, yogurt, avocado, or coconut oil. This can help balance your blood sugar and keep you full longer.

- Drink your juice with a meal or a snack, not on an empty stomach. This can prevent blood sugar spikes and provide more nutrients and fiber from other foods.

- Limit your juice intake to one small glass per day, and drink it slowly. This can help you avoid excess calories and sugar, and savor the flavor and nutrients of your juice.

- Monitor your blood sugar levels before and after drinking juice, and adjust your medication, diet, and exercise accordingly. This can help you prevent hypoglycemia or hyperglycemia, and manage your diabetes better.

IBS Relief: Gut Health and Juicing Strategies

Irritable bowel syndrome (IBS) is a digestive illness that mostly affects the large intestine. It can cause stomach discomfort, bloating, gas, diarrhea, constipation, or a combination of the two. Although the specific etiology of IBS is unknown, it may be connected to stress, nutrition, gut flora, inflammation, or genetics.

Juicing is a process of extracting juice from fruits and vegetables while retaining the majority of the fiber and pulp. Juicing can be an easy method to get extra nutrients, antioxidants, and phytochemicals from plant foods, which may help with gut health and IBS symptoms. However, juicing has significant disadvantages and hazards, particularly for persons with IBS.

In this article, we will discuss the pros and cons of juicing for IBS, and provide some tips and strategies to make juicing safer and healthier for your gut.

Pros of juicing for IBS

- Juicing can help you increase your intake of fruits and vegetables, which are rich in vitamins, minerals, and phytochemicals that can lower inflammation, prevent disease, and promote overall health.

- Juicing can provide some prebiotics, which are types of carbohydrates that feed the beneficial bacteria in your gut and support digestive health. Some examples of prebiotic-rich fruits and vegetables are apples, bananas, berries, asparagus, artichokes, garlic, onion, and leeks.

- Juicing can help you hydrate, as fruits and vegetables have high water content. Staying hydrated can help regulate bowel movements and prevent dehydration, which can worsen IBS symptoms.

- Juicing can help you avoid or reduce your intake of insoluble fiber, which is the type of fiber that adds bulk to stool and helps it pass through the colon. Some people with IBS may be sensitive to insoluble fiber, as it can cause gas, bloating, and abdominal pain. By juicing fruits and vegetables, you are removing most of the insoluble fiber but still getting some of the soluble fiber, which is the type of fiber that dissolves in water and forms a gel-like substance that can soothe the gut and slow down digestion.

Cons of juicing for IBS

- Juicing can raise your blood sugar levels very quickly, as it removes most of the fiber from fruits and vegetables, which slows down the digestion and absorption of carbohydrates. This can lead to spikes and crashes in blood sugar, which can affect your mood, energy, appetite, and insulin sensitivity.

- Juicing can reduce your intake of protein and healthy fats, which are essential for balancing blood sugar, building muscle, and maintaining a healthy weight. Protein and fat also help you feel full and satisfied, which can prevent overeating and cravings.

- Juicing can be expensive, as it requires a lot of fruits and vegetables to make a small amount of juice. It can also be time-consuming and messy, as you need to wash, chop, and juice the produce, and clean the juicer afterwards.

- Juicing can trigger or worsen IBS symptoms in some people, especially if they are sensitive to FODMAPs (fermentable oligosaccharides, disaccharides, monosaccharides, and polyols), which are types of carbohydrates that can cause gas, bloating, and diarrhea in some people with IBS. FODMAPs are found in various amounts in fruits and vegetables, and drinking juices that contain high amounts of FODMAPs may cause IBS flare-ups.

Tips and strategies for juicing with IBS

If you have IBS and want to try juicing, here are some tips and strategies to make it safer and healthier for your gut:

- Choose low-sugar and low-FODMAP fruits and vegetables, such as berries, oranges, grapes, kiwis, pineapple, celery, cucumber, kale, spinach, zucchini, and ginger. Avoid high-sugar and high-FODMAP fruits and vegetables, such as apples, pears, mangoes, watermelon, cherries, peaches, apricots, plums, dates, figs, honey, agave, beetroot, cabbage, cauliflower, broccoli, Brussels sprouts, garlic, onion, and leeks.

- Add some protein and healthy fat to your juice, such as nuts, seeds, yogurt, kefir, tofu, avocado, or coconut oil. This can help balance your blood sugar and keep you full longer.

- Drink your juice with a meal or a snack, not on an empty stomach. This can prevent blood sugar spikes and provide more nutrients and fiber from other foods.

- Limit your juice intake to one small glass per day, and drink it slowly. This can help you avoid excess calories and sugar, and savor the flavor and nutrients of your juice.

- Monitor your blood sugar levels before and after drinking juice, and adjust your medication, diet, and exercise accordingly. This can help you prevent hypoglycemia or hyperglycemia, and manage your diabetes better.

- Keep track of your IBS symptoms and how they relate to your juicing habits. You can use a food diary, an app, or a symptom tracker to record what you eat and drink, when you have IBS symptoms, and how severe they are. This can help you identify your triggers and what works best for you.

Summary

Juicing can have some benefits for people with IBS, such as providing nutrients, antioxidants, and prebiotics, and helping with hydration and insoluble fiber intake. However, juicing can also have some drawbacks and risks, such as raising blood sugar levels, reducing protein and fat intake, and triggering or worsening IBS symptoms in some people. If you have IBS and want to juice, you should choose low-sugar and low-FODMAP fruits and vegetables, add some protein and fat, drink it with a meal or a snack, limit your portion size, and monitor your blood sugar and IBS symptoms. Juicing should not replace a balanced and healthy diet, but rather complement it. Always consult your doctor before making any changes to your diet or medication.

Eczema and Skin Conditions: Nourishing from the Inside Out

Eczema, a chronic inflammatory skin condition, often manifests as red, itchy, and inflamed patches on the skin. While topical treatments can provide relief, addressing eczema from the inside out through proper nutrition is a key component of a holistic approach to skin health. Incorporating specific nutrients and adopting a skin-friendly diet may help manage symptoms and promote overall well-being.

1. Omega-3 Fatty Acids for Skin Integrity: Omega-3 fatty acids, found in fatty fish, flaxseeds, and walnuts, play a crucial role in maintaining skin integrity and reducing inflammation. Including these sources in your diet can contribute to a healthy lipid barrier in the skin, potentially reducing the severity of eczema symptoms.

2. Antioxidant-Rich Fruits and Vegetables: Fruits and vegetables rich in antioxidants, such as berries, citrus fruits, and leafy greens, provide a spectrum of vitamins and minerals that support skin health. Antioxidants combat oxidative stress and free radicals, contributing to a more resilient and radiant complexion.

3. Probiotics for Gut-Health Connection: The gut-skin axis highlights the interconnectedness of gut health and skin conditions. Probiotics, found in yogurt, kefir, and fermented foods, promote a healthy gut microbiome. A balanced gut microbiome may positively influence inflammatory skin conditions like eczema, emphasizing the importance of incorporating probiotic-rich foods into the diet.

4. Vitamin A for Skin Repair: Vitamin A is crucial for skin repair and maintenance. Foods rich in vitamin A, such as sweet potatoes, carrots, and leafy greens, support the regenerative processes of the skin. Adequate vitamin A intake may help mitigate the symptoms of eczema by promoting healthy skin cell turnover.

5. Hydration for Skin Moisture: Maintaining proper hydration is essential for skin health. Drinking an ample amount of water helps keep the skin hydrated from the inside out, reducing dryness and potentially alleviating eczema symptoms. Herbal teas and water-rich fruits like watermelon contribute to overall hydration.

6. Zinc for Wound Healing: Zinc is a mineral crucial for wound healing and skin health. Foods rich in zinc, including pumpkin seeds, chickpeas, and lean meats, support the body's ability to repair damaged skin. Incorporating zinc into the diet may contribute to the overall resilience of the skin barrier.

7. Avoiding Potential Triggers: While nourishing the skin from the inside out is vital, it's equally important to identify and avoid potential dietary triggers that may exacerbate eczema symptoms. Common triggers include certain food allergens, such as dairy, gluten, and nuts. Individual responses vary, so keeping a food diary and consulting with a healthcare professional can aid in identifying specific triggers.

8. Essential Fatty Acids for Skin Moisture: In addition to omega-3 fatty acids, incorporating omega-6 fatty acids from sources like safflower oil, sunflower seeds, and evening primrose oil can help maintain skin moisture. These essential fatty acids contribute to the lipid barrier of the skin, preventing excessive dryness and irritation.

In Conclusion: A holistic approach to managing eczema involves nurturing the skin from the inside out through a balanced and nutrient-dense diet. While dietary changes can be beneficial, it's crucial to consult with healthcare professionals or dermatologists to develop an individualized plan. Combining proper nutrition with other lifestyle adjustments, stress management, and suitable skincare routines creates a comprehensive strategy for promoting skin health and managing eczema symptoms.

Supporting Thyroid Health in Hashimoto's Thyroiditis

Hashimoto's Thyroiditis, an autoimmune condition affecting the thyroid gland, requires a comprehensive approach to support thyroid health and overall well-being. While medical management plays a crucial role, lifestyle factors, including diet, can significantly impact the progression and management of the condition. Adopting a holistic approach that includes specific dietary strategies can be beneficial for individuals dealing with Hashimoto's Thyroiditis.

1. Embracing a Nutrient-Dense Diet: Prioritizing a nutrient-dense diet rich in vitamins, minerals, and antioxidants is essential for supporting thyroid health. Include a variety of whole foods such as fruits, vegetables, lean proteins, and whole grains. These foods provide essential nutrients that contribute to overall well-being and may help alleviate symptoms associated with Hashimoto's Thyroiditis.

2. Incorporating Iodine-Rich Foods in Moderation: Iodine is a crucial component of thyroid hormones, but excessive intake can be detrimental in autoimmune thyroid conditions. While iodine deficiency can impact thyroid function, excessive iodine may exacerbate inflammation in Hashimoto's. Incorporate moderate amounts of iodine-rich foods like seaweed, fish, and dairy, and discuss iodine supplementation with a healthcare professional.

3. Balancing Selenium Intake: Selenium is an essential mineral with antioxidant properties that may help reduce inflammation and support thyroid function. Foods rich in selenium include Brazil nuts, sunflower seeds, and poultry.

Be mindful of selenium intake, aiming for a balance, as excessive amounts can have adverse effects.

4. Prioritizing Gut Health: The gut-thyroid connection is increasingly recognized, and supporting gut health is vital for individuals with autoimmune conditions like Hashimoto's. Include probiotic-rich foods such as yogurt, kefir, and fermented vegetables to promote a healthy gut microbiome. Consider consulting with a healthcare professional about the potential benefits of probiotic supplements.

5. Managing Gluten Intake: Some individuals with Hashimoto's Thyroiditis may experience improvements in symptoms by reducing or eliminating gluten from their diet. Gluten sensitivity is common in autoimmune conditions, and it may contribute to inflammation. Experimenting with a gluten-free diet, under the guidance of a healthcare professional or registered dietitian, can help determine if it positively impacts symptoms.

6. Mindful Consumption of Cruciferous Vegetables: Cruciferous vegetables like broccoli, cauliflower, and kale contain compounds known as goitrogens, which can interfere with thyroid function. However, cooking these vegetables can reduce their goitrogenic effects. Individuals with Hashimoto's may consider incorporating these vegetables into their diet in moderate amounts and preferably cooked.

7. Optimal Hydration and Lifestyle Choices: Staying well-hydrated is crucial for overall health, including thyroid function. Adequate water intake supports metabolic processes and helps maintain optimal bodily functions. Additionally, managing stress through practices like mindfulness, meditation, and adequate sleep is essential, as stress can impact thyroid health and autoimmune conditions.

8. Collaborating with Healthcare Professionals: While dietary strategies play a crucial role, it's important to collaborate with healthcare professionals, including endocrinologists, nutritionists, and other specialists. Regular monitoring of thyroid hormone levels and individualized management plans can ensure comprehensive care tailored to specific needs.

In conclusion, supporting thyroid health in Hashimoto's Thyroiditis involves adopting a holistic approach that integrates dietary strategies with lifestyle choices and medical management. Customizing dietary choices based on individual responses and collaborating closely with healthcare professionals allows for a well-rounded approach to managing symptoms and promoting overall well-being in individuals dealing with Hashimoto's Thyroiditis.

Chapter 3: Customized Juice Healing Plans

Rheumatoid Arthritis Juice Protocol

Rheumatoid Arthritis (RA) is an autoimmune disorder characterized by chronic inflammation of the joints, leading to pain, stiffness, and swelling. While a juice protocol cannot cure RA, certain nutrient-dense ingredients may provide anti-inflammatory and joint-supportive benefits. It's important to note that this protocol is not a substitute for medical treatment, and individuals with RA should consult with healthcare professionals before making significant dietary changes.

1. Anti-Inflammatory Green Elixir: Ingredients:

- 2 cups kale leaves

- 1 cucumber

- 1 green apple

- 1/2 lemon (peeled)

- 1-inch ginger root

Instructions: Juice the kale, cucumber, green apple, lemon, and ginger. This green elixir provides a potent combination of anti-inflammatory compounds, including the anti-inflammatory effects of ginger.

2. Pineapple Turmeric Joint Soother: Ingredients:

- 1 cup pineapple chunks

- 1 inch turmeric root

- 1 carrot

- 1/2 orange (peeled)

Instructions: Juice the pineapple, turmeric, carrot, and orange. Pineapple contains bromelain, known for its anti-inflammatory properties, while turmeric contributes curcumin, a natural anti-inflammatory compound.

3. Ginger Berry Arthritis Buster: Ingredients:

- 1 cup mixed berries (blueberries, strawberries, raspberries)

- 1/2 cucumber

- 1 inch ginger root

- 1/2 lime (peeled)

Instructions: Juice the berries, cucumber, ginger, and lime. Ginger, with its anti-inflammatory and antioxidant properties, complements the antioxidant-rich berries in supporting joint health.

4. Celery Cucumber Hydration Elixir: Ingredients:

- 3 celery stalks

- 1 cucumber

- 1/2 lemon (peeled)

- 1/2 cup parsley

Instructions: Juice the celery, cucumber, lemon, and parsley. Celery provides hydration, while cucumber and parsley contribute anti-inflammatory and antioxidant compounds.

5. Carrot Ginger Joint Comfort Blend: Ingredients:

- 4 carrots

- 1 inch ginger root

- 1 orange (peeled)

- 1/2 turmeric root (optional)

Instructions: Juice the carrots, ginger, orange, and turmeric (if using). Carrots are rich in beta-carotene, and ginger adds anti-inflammatory benefits to support joint comfort.

Tips for Rheumatoid Arthritis Juice Protocol:

1. **Consistency is Key:** Incorporate these juices regularly to maximize potential benefits. However, it's important to maintain a balanced diet and not rely solely on juices.

2. **Consider Dietary Restrictions:** Some individuals with RA may have specific dietary sensitivities or restrictions. Adjust the juice protocol accordingly and consult with a healthcare professional or a registered dietitian.

3. **Stay Hydrated:** Adequate hydration is crucial for joint health. Include water and herbal teas in addition to these juices to support overall hydration.

4. **Monitor Individual Responses:** Pay attention to how your body responds to the juice protocol. If you experience any adverse reactions, consult with healthcare professionals.

5. **Complement with Whole Foods:** While these juices offer concentrated nutrients, a well-rounded diet that includes a variety of whole foods is essential for overall health.

It's crucial to approach the Rheumatoid Arthritis Juice Protocol as part of a holistic management plan that includes medical treatment, exercise, and lifestyle adjustments. Consulting with healthcare professionals ensures a personalized approach that considers individual health needs and potential interactions with medications.

Multiple Sclerosis Wellness Juice Regimen

Multiple Sclerosis (MS) is a chronic autoimmune disease that affects the central nervous system, leading to various symptoms such as fatigue, muscle weakness, and difficulty with coordination. While there is no cure for MS, adopting a wellness-focused lifestyle, including a nutrient-dense juice regimen, may contribute to overall well-being. It's crucial for individuals with MS to consult with healthcare professionals before making significant dietary changes.

1. Neuroprotective Berry Blend: Ingredients:

- 1 cup blueberries
- 1/2 cup strawberries
- 1/2 cup raspberries
- 1 banana (ripe)
- 1/2 cup spinach

Instructions: Blend all ingredients until smooth. Berries are rich in antioxidants, and spinach provides essential nutrients that may support neurological health.

2. Vitamin D Boosting Citrus Elixir: Ingredients:

- 2 oranges (peeled)
- 1/2 grapefruit (peeled)
- 1/2 lemon (peeled)
- 1 carrot
- 1-inch turmeric root (optional)

Instructions: Juice the oranges, grapefruit, lemon, carrot, and turmeric. This elixir provides vitamin D from citrus fruits, which may contribute to immune system support.

3. Anti-Inflammatory Green Detox Juice: Ingredients:

- 2 cups kale leaves

- 1 cucumber

- 1 green apple

- 1/2 lemon (peeled)

- 1-inch ginger root

Instructions: Juice the kale, cucumber, green apple, lemon, and ginger. This green juice offers anti-inflammatory compounds and a refreshing taste.

4. Omega-3 Fatty Acid Brain Booster: Ingredients:

- 1/2 avocado

- 1 cup spinach

- 1/2 cucumber

- 1/2 lime (peeled)

- 1 tablespoon chia seeds

Instructions: Blend the avocado, spinach, cucumber, lime, and chia seeds until smooth. Avocado provides healthy fats, and chia seeds offer omega-3 fatty acids, which are beneficial for brain health.

5. Hydration and Electrolyte Replenisher: Ingredients:

- 1 cup watermelon chunks

- 1 cucumber

- 1/2 lime (peeled)

- Mint leaves for flavor

Instructions: Juice the watermelon, cucumber, and lime. Add mint leaves for flavor. This hydrating juice supports overall hydration and provides natural electrolytes.

Tips for Multiple Sclerosis Wellness Juice Regimen:

1. **Mindful Ingredient Selection:** Choose ingredients rich in antioxidants, vitamins, and minerals that support overall health and may have potential benefits for individuals with MS.

2. **Consider Dietary Sensitivities:** Some individuals with MS may have specific dietary sensitivities. Adjust the juice regimen based on individual needs and consult with healthcare professionals.

3. **Hydration is Key:** Adequate hydration is crucial for individuals with MS. In addition to juices, include water, herbal teas, and water-rich foods in your daily routine.

4. **Monitor Responses:** Pay attention to how your body responds to the juice regimen. If there are any adverse reactions or interactions with medications, consult with healthcare professionals.

5. **Complement with Whole Foods:** While juices offer concentrated nutrients, a balanced diet that includes a variety of whole foods is essential for overall health and wellness.

It's important to approach the Multiple Sclerosis Wellness Juice Regimen as part of a holistic lifestyle that includes medical treatment, regular exercise, and other supportive practices. Consulting with healthcare professionals ensures a personalized approach that considers individual health needs and potential interactions with medications.

Blood Sugar Balance Juice Plan for Type 2 Diabetes

Managing blood sugar levels is crucial for individuals with Type 2 Diabetes, and a well-balanced diet plays a significant role in this process. While whole foods should be the foundation, incorporating nutrient-dense juices can be a complementary part of a diabetes-friendly diet. It's essential for individuals with diabetes to consult with healthcare professionals, including dietitians, before making significant dietary changes.

1. Green Veggie Insulin Regulator: Ingredients:

- 2 cups spinach
- 1 cucumber
- 1 green apple
- 1/2 lemon (peeled)
- 1-inch ginger root

Instructions: Juice the spinach, cucumber, green apple, lemon, and ginger. This green juice provides a mix of vitamins and minerals that may contribute to blood sugar regulation.

2. Citrus Cinnamon Glucose Stabilizer: Ingredients:

- 2 oranges (peeled)
- 1/2 grapefruit (peeled)
- 1/2 lemon (peeled)
- 1 teaspoon ground cinnamon

- 1/2 inch turmeric root (optional)

Instructions: Juice the oranges, grapefruit, and lemon. Add ground cinnamon and turmeric. Cinnamon may have potential benefits for blood sugar balance, and turmeric contributes anti-inflammatory properties.

3. Berry Fiber-Rich Blood Sugar Controller: Ingredients:

- 1 cup blueberries

- 1/2 cup raspberries

- 1/2 cup strawberries

- 1/2 cucumber

- 1 tablespoon chia seeds

Instructions: Juice the berries and cucumber. Stir in chia seeds for added fiber. Berries are low in sugar and high in fiber, supporting blood sugar control.

4. Beta-Carotene Carrot Elixir: Ingredients:

- 4 carrots

- 1/2 orange (peeled)

- 1/2 lemon (peeled)

- 1 inch ginger root

Instructions: Juice the carrots, orange, lemon, and ginger. Carrots provide beta-carotene, and ginger adds a spicy kick with potential anti-inflammatory benefits.

5. Avocado Spinach Blood Sugar Balancer: Ingredients:

- 1/2 avocado

- 1 cup spinach

- 1/2 cucumber

- 1/2 lime (peeled)

- 1 tablespoon flaxseeds

Instructions: Blend the avocado, spinach, cucumber, lime, and flaxseeds. Avocado contributes healthy fats, and flaxseeds add fiber and omega-3 fatty acids.

Tips for Blood Sugar Balance Juice Plan:

1. **Portion Control:** Pay attention to portion sizes and consider the total carbohydrate content of the juices. Balancing macronutrients is crucial for blood sugar management.

2. **Monitor Blood Sugar Levels:** Regularly monitor blood sugar levels to understand how your body responds to different juices. Adjust your plan based on individual responses.

3. **Stay Hydrated:** Alongside juices, ensure adequate hydration with water and herbal teas. Proper hydration supports overall health and can assist in blood sugar regulation.

4. **Include Whole Foods:** While juices can be a valuable addition, whole foods such as vegetables, fruits, lean proteins, and whole grains should form the basis of a diabetes-friendly diet.

5. **Consult with Healthcare Professionals:** Always consult with healthcare professionals, including dietitians and doctors, before making significant

changes to your diet. Individualized advice is crucial for managing diabetes effectively.

It's important to view the Blood Sugar Balance Juice Plan as part of an overall diabetes management strategy that includes medication, regular physical activity, and lifestyle adjustments. Personalized guidance from healthcare professionals ensures that the plan aligns with individual health needs and goals.

IBS Soothing Juice Program

Irritable Bowel Syndrome (IBS) is a common gastrointestinal disorder characterized by symptoms such as abdominal pain, bloating, and changes in bowel habits. While managing IBS involves various strategies, including dietary modifications, a soothing juice program can complement overall gut health. Individuals with IBS should consult with healthcare professionals, including dietitians, before making significant dietary changes.

1. Soothing Aloe Vera Elixir: Ingredients:

- 1 cup fresh aloe vera gel (scoop out from aloe leaves)
- 1 cucumber
- 1 cup coconut water
- 1 tablespoon fresh mint leaves
- 1 tablespoon honey (optional)

Instructions: Blend the aloe vera gel, cucumber, coconut water, mint leaves, and honey. Aloe vera is known for its soothing properties and may provide relief for irritated intestines.

2. Ginger Carrot Digestive Tonic: Ingredients:

- 1-inch ginger root
- 4 carrots
- 1/2 lemon (peeled)
- 1 tablespoon chia seeds (optional)

Instructions: Juice the ginger, carrots, and lemon. Stir in chia seeds if desired. Ginger helps soothe the digestive tract, while carrots contribute essential nutrients for gut health.

3. Gut-Healing Green Smoothie: Ingredients:

- 1 cup spinach

- 1/2 cup Greek yogurt (unsweetened)

- 1 banana (ripe)

- 1/2 cup pineapple chunks

- 1 tablespoon flaxseeds

Instructions: Blend all ingredients until smooth. This green smoothie combines probiotics from yogurt, fiber from spinach, and the digestive benefits of banana and pineapple.

4. Papaya Mint Digestive Elixir: Ingredients:

- 1 cup ripe papaya chunks

- 1 cucumber

- 1/2 lime (peeled)

- Handful of fresh mint leaves

Instructions: Juice the papaya, cucumber, lime, and mint. Papaya contains digestive enzymes, while mint adds a refreshing touch for gastrointestinal comfort.

5. Fennel Pineapple Digestive Tonic: Ingredients:

- 1 cup fennel bulb (sliced)

- 1 cup pineapple chunks

- 1/2 lemon (peeled)

- 1 tablespoon chia seeds (optional)

Instructions: Juice the fennel, pineapple, and lemon. Stir in chia seeds if desired. Fennel's anti-spasmodic properties may help ease digestive discomfort, and pineapple adds natural sweetness.

Tips for IBS Soothing Juice Program:

1. **Start Gradually:** Introduce these juices gradually to assess tolerance and individual responses.

2. **Consider Trigger Foods:** Identify and avoid potential trigger foods that exacerbate IBS symptoms. Common triggers include certain FODMAPs, dairy, and artificial sweeteners.

3. **Stay Hydrated:** Adequate hydration is essential for managing IBS symptoms. Water-rich fruits and vegetables in the juices contribute to overall hydration.

4. **Monitor Portion Sizes:** Be mindful of portion sizes to avoid overwhelming the digestive system. Smaller, frequent servings may be more comfortable.

5. **Seek Professional Guidance:** Consult with healthcare professionals, including dietitians, to create an individualized IBS management plan. They can provide personalized advice based on your specific needs and triggers.

6. **Combine with Lifestyle Adjustments:** In addition to the juice program, consider lifestyle modifications such as stress management, regular physical activity, and sufficient sleep for comprehensive IBS management.

The IBS Soothing Juice Program is meant to be part of an overall strategy for managing IBS symptoms. It's important to understand individual triggers and preferences while seeking guidance from healthcare professionals for a tailored approach to gut health.

Eczema Healing Elixirs

Eczema is a chronic inflammatory skin condition characterized by red, itchy, and inflamed patches. While topical treatments are essential, addressing eczema from within through a nourishing diet can complement external skincare efforts. These healing elixirs incorporate ingredients known for their potential benefits in supporting skin health. Individuals with eczema should consult with healthcare professionals, including dermatologists and nutritionists, before making significant dietary changes.

1. Omega-3 Rich Berry Bliss: Ingredients:

- 1 cup mixed berries (blueberries, strawberries, raspberries)

- 1/2 avocado

- 1 tablespoon chia seeds

- 1 cup almond milk (unsweetened)

Instructions: Blend the mixed berries, avocado, chia seeds, and almond milk until smooth. This elixir provides omega-3 fatty acids from chia seeds and healthy fats from avocado to support skin hydration and reduce inflammation.

2. Anti-Inflammatory Turmeric Gold Elixir: Ingredients:

- 1-inch turmeric root

- 1/2 pineapple (peeled and cored)

- 1/2 cucumber

- 1 tablespoon honey (optional)

- 1 cup coconut water

Instructions: Juice the turmeric, pineapple, and cucumber. Stir in honey if desired and mix with coconut water. Turmeric's anti-inflammatory properties may help alleviate eczema symptoms, while pineapple adds natural sweetness.

3. Probiotic Green Gut Soother: Ingredients:

- 1 cup spinach

- 1/2 cucumber

- 1/2 banana (ripe)

- 1/2 cup Greek yogurt (unsweetened)

- 1/2 lime (peeled)

Instructions: Blend the spinach, cucumber, banana, Greek yogurt, and lime until smooth. This green elixir combines gut-friendly probiotics from yogurt with the skin-soothing benefits of spinach.

4. Vitamin C Citrus Radiance Tonic: Ingredients:

- 1 orange (peeled)

- 1/2 grapefruit (peeled)

- 1/2 lemon (peeled)

- 1 tablespoon flaxseeds

- 1 cup water

Instructions: Juice the orange, grapefruit, and lemon. Blend with flaxseeds and water. This vitamin C-rich tonic supports collagen production and may aid in skin repair.

5. Hydrating Cucumber Mint Cooler: Ingredients:

- 1 cucumber

- Handful of fresh mint leaves

- 1/2 lime (peeled)

- 1 tablespoon aloe vera gel

- 1 cup coconut water

Instructions: Juice the cucumber, mint, and lime. Stir in aloe vera gel and mix with coconut water. This hydrating cooler incorporates aloe vera for its soothing properties and mint for a refreshing flavor.

Tips for Eczema Healing Elixirs:

1. **Individualize Ingredients:** Be aware of personal triggers and sensitivities. Adjust the elixir recipes based on individual responses.

2. **Stay Hydrated:** Proper hydration is essential for skin health. Incorporate water-rich ingredients and ensure sufficient overall fluid intake.

3. **Monitor Sugar Intake:** Limit added sugars, as excessive sugar consumption may contribute to inflammation. Choose naturally sweet ingredients instead.

4. **Consistency is Key:** Include these elixirs regularly as part of a balanced diet to potentially see skin-improving benefits over time.

5. **Seek Professional Advice:** Consult with healthcare professionals, especially dermatologists and nutritionists, for personalized guidance on managing eczema through diet and skincare.

Remember that while these elixirs may provide potential benefits, they should be part of a comprehensive approach to eczema management, including proper skincare, avoiding known triggers, and consulting with healthcare professionals for tailored advice.

Thyroid Supportive Juices for Hashimoto's Thyroiditis

Hashimoto's Thyroiditis is an autoimmune condition affecting the thyroid gland, leading to inflammation and potential disruption of thyroid function. While juice alone cannot replace medical treatment, incorporating thyroid-supportive ingredients into your diet may contribute to overall thyroid health. Individuals with Hashimoto's should consult with healthcare professionals, including endocrinologists and nutritionists, for personalized advice before making significant dietary changes.

1. Thyroid-Boosting Green Elixir: Ingredients:

- 2 cups kale leaves
- 1 cucumber
- 1 green apple
- 1/2 lemon (peeled)
- 1-inch ginger root

Instructions: Juice the kale, cucumber, green apple, lemon, and ginger. This green elixir provides a wealth of vitamins and minerals that may support thyroid function, with ginger offering anti-inflammatory properties.

2. Iodine-Balancing Sea Greens Juice: Ingredients:

- 1/2 cup seaweed (dulse or nori)
- 1 cucumber
- 1 carrot

- 1/2 lemon (peeled)

Instructions: Juice the seaweed, cucumber, carrot, and lemon. Seaweed is a natural source of iodine, a vital component of thyroid hormones, contributing to a balanced thyroid function.

3. Antioxidant-Rich Berry Thyroid Tonic: Ingredients:

- 1 cup mixed berries (blueberries, strawberries, raspberries)
- 1/2 avocado
- 1 tablespoon chia seeds
- 1/2 lime (peeled)

Instructions: Blend the mixed berries, avocado, chia seeds, and lime until smooth. Berries provide antioxidants, while avocado contributes healthy fats beneficial for thyroid health.

4. Selenium-Infused Citrus Elixir: Ingredients:

- 2 oranges (peeled)
- 1/2 grapefruit (peeled)
- 1 Brazil nut (for selenium)
- 1/2 lemon (peeled)

Instructions: Juice the oranges, grapefruit, and lemon. Incorporate a whole Brazil nut for its selenium content, a mineral crucial for thyroid function.

5. Thyroid-Supportive Carrot Ginger Elixir: Ingredients:

- 4 carrots

- 1 inch ginger root

- 1 orange (peeled)

- 1/2 turmeric root (optional)

Instructions: Juice the carrots, ginger, orange, and turmeric (if using). Carrots provide beta-carotene, and ginger adds anti-inflammatory benefits to support thyroid health.

Tips for Thyroid Supportive Juices:

1. **Moderation is Key:** While iodine and selenium are essential, excessive intake may have adverse effects. Consult with healthcare professionals to determine appropriate levels for your individual needs.

2. **Consistency Matters:** Include these juices regularly as part of a balanced diet. Consistency over time may contribute to potential thyroid-supportive benefits.

3. **Individualize Ingredients:** Pay attention to your body's responses and adjust ingredient quantities based on individual sensitivities or preferences.

4. **Complement with Whole Foods:** Juices should be part of a comprehensive approach. Include a variety of whole foods rich in nutrients supporting overall health and thyroid function.

5. **Monitor Thyroid Levels:** Regularly monitor thyroid hormone levels through blood tests, and work closely with healthcare professionals to manage Hashimoto's Thyroiditis effectively.

While these thyroid-supportive juices may offer potential benefits, they should be viewed as part of a broader strategy that includes medical management, a well-balanced diet, and lifestyle considerations. Consulting with healthcare professionals ensures a personalized approach aligned with individual health needs and goals.

Chapter 4: Integrating Juicing into Daily Life

Creating Sustainable Habits: Juicing as a Lifestyle

Juicing, when approached as a lifestyle, offers a gateway to sustainable and health-conscious habits. The key to integrating juicing into daily life lies in fostering a balanced and realistic approach that considers individual preferences, nutritional needs, and long-term wellness goals. The first step in creating sustainable juicing habits is to view it as a complement to a diverse and nutrient-rich diet. Rather than relying solely on juices, they should be incorporated alongside whole foods, ensuring a broad spectrum of essential nutrients. This not only enhances the nutritional profile but also prevents potential drawbacks associated with excessive sugar intake from fruit-heavy juices.

Building sustainable juicing habits involves cultivating mindfulness around ingredient selection. Prioritizing seasonal, locally sourced produce not only supports environmental sustainability but also provides access to fresher and more nutrient-dense ingredients. This approach aligns juicing with broader principles of conscious consumption and encourages a connection with the local food ecosystem. Additionally, varying the ingredients regularly helps prevent monotony, keeping the habit enjoyable and preventing flavor fatigue.

A crucial aspect of sustainable juicing is to acknowledge individual preferences and dietary requirements. Customizing juice recipes based on taste preferences and nutritional needs fosters a sense of ownership and enjoyment in the process. Including a mix of fruits, vegetables, and functional ingredients like ginger or turmeric adds diversity in flavor and health benefits. This adaptability ensures that juicing remains an adaptable and enjoyable part of daily life, rather than a restrictive or monotonous routine.

To make juicing sustainable, it's essential to consider practical aspects of lifestyle. Investing in a high-quality juicer that aligns with personal preferences, whether it's a slow masticating juicer for nutrient retention or a convenient centrifugal one for quick preparations, enhances the overall experience. Moreover, planning and preparing ingredients ahead of time can save valuable minutes in a busy schedule, making juicing a feasible and time-efficient choice.

Creating sustainable juicing habits also involves recognizing the role of hydration in overall well-being. Juices, enriched with water-rich fruits and vegetables, contribute to daily fluid intake. This dual benefit not only supports hydration but also aids in the absorption of vital nutrients. Incorporating herbal teas and water alongside juices ensures a holistic approach to staying well-hydrated.

Beyond the physical aspect, sustainability in juicing extends to the mental and emotional dimensions of well-being.

Establishing a positive relationship with juicing involves embracing it as a tool for self-care rather than a strict regimen. Setting realistic goals, celebrating small achievements, and allowing flexibility in the juicing routine fosters a positive mindset. It's crucial to view juicing not as a temporary fix but as a lifelong journey towards optimal health.

In conclusion, making juicing a sustainable lifestyle involves a holistic and mindful approach that integrates seamlessly with individual preferences and daily routines. By embracing diversity in ingredients, prioritizing local and seasonal produce, investing in quality equipment, and maintaining a positive mindset, juicing becomes a nourishing and enjoyable habit. Ultimately, the sustainable juicing lifestyle is not just about what goes into the juicer but also about cultivating a mindful and balanced approach to well-being that extends far beyond the kitchen.

Tips for Incorporating Juices into Meals

Incorporating juices into meals can be a delightful way to enhance the nutritional content of your diet. Here are some tips to seamlessly integrate juices into your meals:

1. **Pair with Balanced Meals:**

   - Consider juices as complementary components of a well-rounded meal. Include a mix of proteins, carbohydrates, and healthy fats alongside your juice to create a balanced and satisfying plate.

2. **Use Juices as Refreshing Starters:**

   - Begin your meal with a small glass of freshly squeezed juice. This not only provides a burst of vitamins and minerals but also serves as a refreshing and hydrating prelude to your main course.

3. **Create Juice-Based Sauces or Dressings:**

   - Use juice as a base for sauces or dressings. For instance, a citrus-based dressing can add zing to salads, or a tomato-based juice can be a flavorful foundation for pasta sauces.

4. **Blend into Smoothie Bowls:**

   - Incorporate juices into smoothie bowls by using them as the liquid base. Blend your favorite fruits and vegetables with yogurt or plant-based alternatives for a nutritious and vibrant meal.

5. **Make Juicy Popsicles:**

- Freeze your favorite juices in popsicle molds. These frozen treats can serve as a refreshing and healthy dessert or snack, adding a burst of flavor to your meals.

6. **Mix with Nutrient-Dense Ingredients:**

   - Boost the nutritional content of your juices by adding nutrient-dense ingredients like chia seeds, flaxseeds, or even a handful of greens. This not only enhances the health benefits but also adds texture and variety.

7. **Pair with Lean Proteins:**

   - Combine juices with lean protein sources such as grilled chicken, fish, or tofu. The natural sweetness of the juice can complement the savory flavors of protein, creating a well-balanced dish.

8. **Experiment with Soup Bases:**

   - Use vegetable-based juices as a base for soups. This adds depth of flavor and nutritional richness to your soups, making them both delicious and nourishing.

9. **Create Colorful Salad Dressings:**

   - Mix fruit-based juices with olive oil, herbs, and seasonings to create vibrant and flavorful salad dressings. Drizzle these over your favorite salads for an extra nutritional boost.

10. **Integrate into Breakfast:**

- Start your day with a nutrient-packed juice alongside your breakfast. Whether it's a green juice with eggs or a fruit-infused smoothie with oats, this sets a positive tone for the rest of the day.

11. **Experiment with Mocktails:**

- Create non-alcoholic mocktails by combining juices with sparkling water or herbal teas. These can serve as refreshing beverages that complement your meals.

12. **Serve as a Palette Cleanser:**

- Use a small glass of juice between courses as a palate cleanser. This can refresh your taste buds and enhance the overall dining experience.

Remember to personalize these tips based on your taste preferences and dietary needs. By getting creative and experimenting with different combinations, you can easily incorporate the goodness of juices into your meals, making them both nutritious and enjoyable.

Overcoming Challenges and Staying Consistent

Embarking on any transformative journey, whether it's adopting a healthier lifestyle, cultivating new habits, or pursuing personal goals, comes with its set of challenges. One key factor in achieving long-term success is navigating these challenges with resilience and maintaining consistency. One significant hurdle is the initial adjustment period, where the novelty of change may wear off, and the allure of old habits can be tempting. During this phase, it's essential to anchor your motivation in a deeper understanding of the reasons behind your pursuit, creating a sustainable source of inspiration that transcends fleeting motivations.

Another common challenge is the pressure of perfectionism, the belief that every step must be flawless. Overcoming this obstacle involves embracing imperfection and viewing setbacks as opportunities for growth rather than failures. Recognizing that setbacks are part of any journey allows for a more forgiving and positive mindset. Additionally, setting realistic expectations and breaking down larger goals into manageable steps can make the path forward less daunting, fostering a sense of accomplishment along the way.

External factors, such as time constraints and competing priorities, can also pose challenges. Effectively managing time and creating a supportive environment are crucial. This may involve strategic planning, delegating tasks, or enlisting the support of friends and family. Establishing a routine that aligns with your goals and allows for flexibility enables a more sustainable and adaptive approach to consistency.

Social influences and societal norms can present challenges, especially when they conflict with personal choices. Staying true to your path often requires navigating external expectations and forging your unique journey. Cultivating a strong sense of self-awareness and resilience helps withstand external pressures, allowing you to remain authentic to your goals.

In the pursuit of consistency, mindset plays a pivotal role. Developing a growth mindset, where challenges are seen as opportunities to learn and improve, fosters resilience. Viewing setbacks as temporary rather than insurmountable encourages perseverance. Mindfulness practices, such as meditation or journaling, can aid in cultivating a positive and resilient mindset, serving as a valuable anchor during challenging times.

Celebrating small victories along the way contributes significantly to sustaining momentum. Acknowledging progress, no matter how incremental, reinforces the sense of achievement and motivates further action. Additionally, building a support network, whether through friends, family, or online communities, provides encouragement and accountability, making the journey less solitary and more empowering.

The ebb and flow of motivation is a natural aspect of any transformative journey. To counteract periods of low motivation, incorporating elements of enjoyment and passion into the process is crucial. Finding joy in the pursuit of your goals, whether it's through discovering new aspects of a healthy lifestyle, relishing the learning process, or appreciating the positive impact on well-being, can rekindle enthusiasm and commitment.

Ultimately, staying consistent amidst challenges is an ongoing process that requires adaptability, self-compassion, and a steadfast commitment to personal growth. Embracing challenges as integral parts of the journey, fostering a resilient mindset, and finding joy in the pursuit can transform obstacles into stepping stones towards lasting success. By approaching challenges with perseverance and cultivating sustainable habits, individuals can navigate the complexities of their journey and realize the fulfillment of their aspirations.

Chapter 5: Success Stories and Testimonials

Inspiring Journeys of Healing through Juicing

In a bustling world filled with various demands and stressors, many individuals have embarked on inspiring journeys of healing through the simple yet profound act of juicing. Take, for example, a person who, amidst the chaos of a demanding job and a sedentary lifestyle, found solace in the vibrant colors of fresh fruits and vegetables. Struggling with energy slumps and a general sense of malaise, they turned to juicing as a way to infuse their body with essential nutrients.

Another relatable story involves someone navigating the complexities of managing a chronic condition. Faced with the challenges of traditional treatments and seeking complementary approaches, they discovered the potential healing power of juicing. Incorporating anti-inflammatory ingredients and immune-boosting fruits, this individual found a renewed sense of vitality and resilience in the face of health challenges.

Consider someone who is experiencing stress and anxiety in terms of emotional well-being. Juicing became a kind of self-care for them on their path of self-discovery. The ritual of choosing, cooking, and tasting fresh food evolved into a therapeutic practice, providing moments of awareness among life's pressures. The brilliant colors and tastes reflected their happy mental and emotional condition, establishing a stronger connection to inner serenity.

A relatable scenario involves a family aiming to instill healthy habits in their daily routine. With busy schedules and the allure of processed snacks, parents sought a way to encourage their children to embrace nutritious choices. Juicing became a family affair, transforming kitchen time into a collaborative and educational experience. The children, once hesitant about vegetables, embraced the colorful concoctions, and the act of juicing became a symbol of shared well-being.

In all these inspiring journeys, the essence lies not just in the act of juicing itself but in the transformative power it holds. It's a process that extends beyond the kitchen, touching various facets of life. These relatable narratives showcase the universal nature of seeking healing, balance, and well-being. Through juicing, individuals find a tangible and accessible means to reconnect with their health, demonstrating that the journey to healing is a personal, evolving, and often beautiful story.

Real-life Experiences: Triumphs and Transformations

In the tapestry of real-life experiences, stories of triumphs and transformations emerge as testaments to the resilience of the human spirit. Consider a professional navigating the competitive landscape of their industry, grappling with the pressure of deadlines and the relentless pursuit of success. Amidst the hustle, they found themselves drained, both mentally and physically. Recognizing the need for a holistic approach to well-being, they turned to juicing as a practical solution.

Embracing a lifestyle centered around nutrient-dense juices became a strategic choice, enhancing their energy levels and cognitive function. This individual discovered that the act of nourishing the body with fresh and vibrant ingredients not only revitalized their professional performance but also became a cornerstone for mental clarity and sustained focus. The triumph here lies not just in career success but in the profound transformation of overall well-being.

Another real-life scenario involves a professional athlete navigating the demanding rigors of training and recovery. In their pursuit of peak performance, they integrated juicing into their regimen. The goal was not only to replenish essential nutrients lost during intense workouts but also to harness the anti-inflammatory properties of specific ingredients. This athlete's journey reflects a triumph over physical limitations and a transformative shift towards a more sustainable and health-conscious approach to their athletic career.

In the corporate world, where burnout and stress are prevalent, a business executive found solace in the rejuvenating power of juicing. Battling the adverse effects of a high-stakes environment, this individual turned to a daily ritual of blending fresh fruits and vegetables. The tangible impact was evident in increased resilience, improved mood, and enhanced clarity in decision-making. The triumph here lies in the ability to navigate a high-stress environment while maintaining a focus on holistic well-being.

Within these real-life experiences, the common thread is the recognition that triumphs and transformations are often rooted in intentional, health-oriented choices. Juicing serves as a tangible catalyst for positive change, fostering not only physical well-being but also mental acuity and emotional resilience. These real and professional narratives illustrate that the journey toward triumph and transformation is ongoing, marked by deliberate choices that contribute to a more balanced and fulfilling life.

Chapter 6: Beyond Juicing: Holistic Approaches to Wellness

Exercise and Movement for Disease Management

Engaging in regular exercise and movement is a cornerstone of holistic health, playing a pivotal role in the management of various diseases. From cardiovascular conditions to metabolic disorders, arthritis, and mental health issues, the positive impact of physical activity on overall well-being is well-documented. This comprehensive approach extends beyond the conventional view of exercise solely as a means for weight management, delving into its multifaceted benefits for disease prevention, symptom alleviation, and overall quality of life.

1. Cardiovascular Health: Regular aerobic exercise, such as walking, jogging, or cycling, is instrumental in maintaining cardiovascular health. For individuals managing conditions like hypertension or heart disease, cardiovascular exercise contributes to improved blood circulation, lowered blood pressure, and enhanced heart function. It also aids in the reduction of LDL cholesterol and triglycerides, mitigating the risk of cardiovascular events.

2. Metabolic Conditions: For those grappling with metabolic disorders like diabetes, exercise emerges as a potent tool. Physical activity enhances insulin sensitivity, promoting better blood sugar control. Incorporating a mix of aerobic exercises and resistance training not only helps manage existing conditions but also aids in the prevention of type 2 diabetes by maintaining a healthy body weight and optimizing insulin function.

3. Musculoskeletal Disorders: In the realm of musculoskeletal disorders such as arthritis, tailored exercise regimens prove invaluable. Low-impact activities like swimming or yoga help improve joint flexibility, reduce pain, and enhance overall mobility. Strength training further supports joint stability, preventing further deterioration and fostering an improved quality of life for individuals managing these conditions.

4. Mental Health and Neurological Disorders: Beyond the physical realm, exercise is a powerful ally in managing mental health conditions and neurological disorders. Regular physical activity releases endorphins, the body's natural mood lifters, contributing to reduced symptoms of depression and anxiety. Additionally, for individuals with neurodegenerative conditions like Parkinson's or Alzheimer's, certain forms of exercise show promise in slowing cognitive decline and improving overall brain health.

5. Respiratory Conditions: Individuals managing respiratory conditions, such as chronic obstructive pulmonary disease (COPD) or asthma, benefit from targeted exercises that enhance lung capacity and respiratory function. Breathing exercises, coupled with aerobic activities tailored to individual capacities, can improve respiratory efficiency and contribute to a better quality of life.

6. Cancer Survivorship: For cancer survivors, incorporating regular exercise into their routine has shown positive outcomes in managing fatigue, improving mood, and reducing the risk of recurrence. Tailored exercise programs, designed in collaboration with healthcare professionals, contribute to the overall well-being of individuals post-cancer treatment.

7. Holistic Well-being: The holistic benefits of exercise extend to stress management, sleep improvement, and enhanced immune function. Engaging in physical activity fosters a sense of accomplishment and empowerment, crucial elements in the overall journey of disease management.

In adopting a holistic approach to well-being, individuals are encouraged to consult with healthcare professionals to tailor exercise programs to their specific needs and conditions. Whether through individualized physical therapy, group classes, or self-guided routines, the integration of regular exercise and movement emerges as a dynamic and empowering strategy in the comprehensive management of various diseases. The journey towards better health is often a blend of medical interventions, lifestyle modifications, and the transformative power of intentional movement.

Stress Management and Mind-Body Connection

In the intricate tapestry of our lives, stress often weaves its threads, affecting our mental and physical well-being. Stress, in its various forms, can manifest as a relentless force, impacting everything from our emotions to our bodily functions. Acknowledging this intricate dance between the mind and body is fundamental to effective stress management. The mind-body connection, a concept deeply rooted in ancient practices like yoga and meditation, has gained substantial recognition in contemporary wellness discourse. It reflects the intricate interplay between our thoughts, emotions, and physiological responses, highlighting the profound influence each realm exerts on the other.

Central to stress management is the cultivation of mindfulness—a practice that encourages us to be fully present in the current moment. Mindfulness serves as a gentle guide, helping individuals navigate the complexities of their thoughts and emotions with a non-judgmental awareness. Techniques such as deep breathing, progressive muscle relaxation, and meditation become invaluable tools in fostering a harmonious mind-body connection. Through these practices, individuals can witness the ebb and flow of stress, gaining insights into its triggers and learning to respond with resilience.

Physical activity, another cornerstone of stress management, acts as a bridge between the mind and body. Exercise releases endorphins, the body's natural mood elevators, fostering a sense of well-being. Beyond the physiological benefits, regular physical activity becomes a mindful practice when approached with intention. Whether through the rhythmic cadence of a jog, the deliberate movements of yoga, or the grace of tai chi, individuals synchronize their mental and physical states, forging a deeper connection between the two.

Nutrition, often underestimated in its role in stress management, is a potent influencer of the mind-body connection. The foods we consume can impact neurotransmitter production, hormonal balance, and overall brain function. A diet rich in whole foods, including fruits, vegetables, and omega-3 fatty acids, nurtures not only the body but also supports cognitive function and emotional well-being. Conversely, excessive intake of processed foods, caffeine, and refined sugars can contribute to inflammation and heightened stress responses. Thus, mindful eating becomes a vital component of fostering a balanced mind-body connection.

Cultivating social connections forms another layer of the mind-body symphony. Human beings, inherently social creatures, thrive on positive interactions and a sense of belonging. Meaningful relationships offer emotional support, reducing the physiological and psychological toll of stress. Sharing experiences, seeking empathy, and offering a listening ear create a harmonious exchange that reverberates through the mind and body.

In the realm of holistic well-being, practices like acupuncture and massage therapy emerge as therapeutic modalities that bridge the mind-body gap. Acupuncture, rooted in traditional Chinese medicine, involves the insertion of thin needles into specific points on the body to restore the flow of energy. Massage therapy, on the other hand, utilizes touch to release muscle tension, promote relaxation, and enhance overall well-being. Both approaches recognize the interconnectedness of physical and mental states, providing avenues for individuals to release physical tension and promote mental calm.

In essence, stress management becomes an art of integration, where the mind and body coalesce in a dance of awareness and self-care. By nurturing the mind-body connection, individuals embark on a transformative journey towards holistic well-being. Each breath, every mindful step, and the conscious choice of nourishment become threads in the tapestry of a balanced, resilient, and harmonious existence. In this symphony of self-care, stress finds its counterpoint, and individuals discover the power to navigate life's challenges with grace and equilibrium.

Sleep, Hydration, and Additional Lifestyle Considerations

Sleep: The Restorative Pillar of Well-being

In the pursuit of holistic well-being, sleep stands as a foundational pillar, wielding profound implications for physical, mental, and emotional health. Adequate and restful sleep is not merely a luxury; it is a vital process during which the body undergoes essential restoration and repair. Sleep plays a pivotal role in cognitive function, memory consolidation, and emotional resilience. The circadian rhythm, often referred to as the body's internal clock, regulates various physiological processes during sleep, influencing hormone release, immune function, and cellular repair. Prioritizing consistent and quality sleep fosters a resilient foundation for navigating the challenges of daily life, contributing to enhanced overall well-being.

Hydration: Nourishing the Body's Vital Functions

Hydration, seemingly straightforward yet profoundly impactful, is a fundamental element of holistic health. The human body, comprising about 60% water, relies on this essential fluid for a myriad of vital functions. Adequate hydration supports digestion, nutrient absorption, and the regulation of body temperature. It plays a crucial role in maintaining skin health, joint lubrication, and overall cellular function. Beyond the physical realm, hydration influences cognitive function and concentration. As a cornerstone of well-being, staying adequately hydrated is not merely about quenching thirst; it is about nourishing the body at a cellular level, promoting optimal function, and creating a hydrated canvas for overall health.

Additional Lifestyle Considerations: Crafting a Holistic Mosaic

Beyond the fundamental elements of sleep and hydration, additional lifestyle considerations intricately weave into the fabric of holistic well-being. A balanced and diverse diet, rich in nutrients, fuels the body with the energy necessary for daily activities and supports long-term health. Regular physical activity, tailored to individual preferences and needs, not only enhances cardiovascular health but also contributes to mental clarity, emotional balance, and overall vitality. Mindful practices, such as meditation, deep-breathing exercises, or yoga, serve as anchors amidst the hustle of daily life, fostering stress management and resilience. Social connections, the quality of relationships, the pursuit of passions, and the cultivation of a positive mindset are essential threads in the intricate mosaic of well-being. Recognizing and embracing the interconnected nature of these lifestyle considerations enables individuals to embark on a transformative journey toward comprehensive health, where each element harmoniously complements the others, creating a resilient and flourishing tapestry of well-being.

Chapter 7: Cooking with Juicer Pulp: Reducing Waste, Maximizing Nutrition

Creative Recipes Using Leftover Juicer Pulp

The aftermath of juicing often leaves behind a bounty of nutrient-rich pulp, bursting with flavors and potential. Rather than consigning this fiber-packed goodness to the compost, let's explore a myriad of creative recipes that transform leftover juicer pulp into culinary delights.

1. Fiber-Packed Veggie Patties:

Transforming leftover juicer pulp into savory veggie patties is a culinary adventure that combines nutrition and taste. Begin by mixing the pulp with cooked quinoa, chickpea flour, and an array of aromatic spices such as cumin, coriander, and paprika. The pulp, rich in fiber and nutrients, adds both texture and flavor to the patties. Form the mixture into patties and pan-fry until golden brown on both sides. The result is a delightful veggie patty that can be served as a protein-packed sandwich filling or as the star of a vibrant salad. These patties not only offer a unique way to repurpose pulp but also introduce a burst of plant-based goodness to your meals.

2. Pulp-Powered Pasta Sauce:

Elevate your pasta dishes by incorporating leftover juicer pulp into a homemade sauce that is both wholesome and flavorful. Combine the pulp with fresh tomatoes, garlic, onions, and a medley of your favorite herbs such as basil and oregano. Simmer the mixture until it transforms into a rich and hearty pasta sauce. The pulp, infused with the essence of various vegetables, adds depth and nutritional value to the sauce. Pour it over your favorite pasta for a meal that not only satisfies your taste buds but also ensures that no valuable nutrients go to waste. This innovative pasta sauce offers a delicious solution to utilizing leftover pulp in a way that complements your favorite Italian dishes.

3. Crunchy Pulp Granola:

Give your mornings a nutritious and crunchy boost by repurposing fruit pulp into a homemade granola. Combine the fruit pulp with oats, nuts, seeds, and a drizzle of maple syrup or honey. Spread the mixture on a baking sheet and bake until golden brown, stirring occasionally for an even crunch. The result is a flavorful and fiber-rich granola that can be used as a topping for yogurt, paired with milk, or enjoyed as a standalone snack. This inventive use of pulp not only reduces waste but also adds a layer of natural sweetness and texture to your breakfast routine. The granola becomes a delicious way to kick-start your day with a blend of wholesome ingredients that might have otherwise been discarded.

4. Fruity Pulp Muffins:

Give your traditional muffin recipe a nutritious twist by incorporating leftover fruit pulp. Whether it's carrot, apple, or mixed berry pulp, these fruity additions bring natural sweetness and moisture to your muffins. Start by preparing your favorite muffin batter, and then fold in the fruit pulp until well combined. The pulp not only enhances the flavor but also contributes additional fiber and vitamins. Bake the muffins until golden brown and enjoy a delightful treat that makes the most of your juicing remnants. These pulp-infused muffins offer a creative way to enjoy a burst of fruity goodness in a convenient and portable form, perfect for breakfast or as a snack.

5. Pulp-Packed Smoothie Bowls:

Take your morning smoothie bowls to the next level by incorporating leftover fruit pulp. Blend the pulp with frozen fruits, yogurt, and a splash of nut milk to create a thick and luscious smoothie base. Pour the smoothie into a bowl and top it with granola, nuts, and fresh fruit for added texture and flavor. This innovative use of pulp not only reduces waste but also transforms your regular smoothie into a more substantial and visually appealing dish. The diverse textures and flavors of the pulp-infused smoothie bowl make it a satisfying and nutritious breakfast option that celebrates the vibrant remnants of your juicing endeavors.

6. Zero-Waste Veggie Broth:

Turn leftover vegetable pulp into a zero-waste vegetable broth that forms the basis for hearty soups, stews, and risottos. Collect and freeze vegetable pulp over time, including scraps like carrot ends, onion peels, and celery leaves. When you have a substantial amount, simmer the frozen pulp with water, garlic, herbs, and seasoning to create a rich and flavorful broth. Strain the liquid to remove solids, leaving you with a nutritious broth that enhances the depth of flavor in your culinary creations. This zero-waste approach not only maximizes the nutritional value of the vegetables but also contributes to sustainable and mindful cooking practices.

7. Pulp-Based Veggie Fritters:

Transform leftover vegetable pulp into delectable and crispy veggie fritters that make for a delightful side dish or snack. Begin by combining the pulp with grated potatoes, breadcrumbs, and an assortment of aromatic spices. Form the mixture into patties and pan-fry until golden brown and crispy on the outside. These veggie fritters not only provide a burst of flavor but also offer a creative way to repurpose pulp into a satisfying and savory treat. Serve them with a dipping sauce or as a complement to a larger meal, showcasing the versatility of juicer pulp in crafting appetizing and nutritious dishes.

8. Pulp-Infused Hummus:

Elevate the classic hummus by incorporating vegetable pulp into the traditional chickpea mixture. The pulp adds a unique texture and an extra layer of flavor, making your homemade hummus a vibrant and nutrient-rich dip. Combine chickpeas, tahini, lemon juice, garlic, and olive oil with the vegetable pulp in a food processor, blending until smooth. The result is a colorful and flavorful hummus that can be enjoyed with fresh veggies, pita bread, or as a spread in sandwiches. This innovative use of pulp not only enhances the nutritional profile of the hummus but also adds a touch of creativity to a beloved and versatile dish.

9. Pulp-Powered Energy Bites:

Craft wholesome and nutritious energy bites by combining fruit pulp with oats, nuts, and a drizzle of honey. Mix the ingredients until well combined, then roll the mixture into bite-sized balls. These energy bites serve as a convenient and satisfying snack that provides a natural sweetness from the fruit pulp and a boost of energy from the wholesome ingredients. Whether enjoyed as a post-workout treat or an afternoon pick-me-up, these pulp-powered energy bites showcase a delicious and efficient way to repurpose juicer remnants into a nutritious and portable snack.

10. Pulp-Based Ice Pops:

Beat the heat with homemade ice pops that incorporate leftover fruit pulp for a refreshing and guilt-free treat. Mix the pulp with coconut water or fruit juice, pour the mixture into molds, and freeze until solid. The result is a colorful and flavorful ice pop that captures the essence of the juiced fruits. These homemade treats not only offer a delightful way to cool down but also reduce waste by utilizing every bit of the juicer remnants. Whether enjoyed by kids and adults alike, these pulp-based ice pops provide a fun and creative solution to turning leftover pulp into a summertime favorite.

Sustainable and Nutrient-Rich Culinary Innovations

1. Utilizing Leftover Juicer Pulp: Embracing sustainability in the kitchen has sparked a culinary revolution, with innovative uses for leftover juicer pulp leading the way. Rather than discarding this fiber-packed byproduct, creative chefs and home cooks have discovered a plethora of ways to repurpose it. From fiber-packed veggie patties and fruity muffins to zero-waste vegetable broth and pulp-infused hummus, these ingenious culinary creations not only minimize food waste but also elevate the nutritional content of meals. This approach not only aligns with eco-conscious practices but also introduces a burst of flavors and textures that add depth and vibrancy to dishes.

2. Redefining Nutrient-Packed Breakfasts: The breakfast table has become a canvas for redefining nutrient-packed morning rituals. From crunchy pulp granola, which transforms juicer remnants into a wholesome topping, to pulp-packed smoothie bowls that turn breakfast into a colorful and nutrient-rich experience, culinary innovators are breathing new life into the first meal of the day. These creations not only ensure a boost of essential vitamins and minerals but also infuse mornings with a burst of creativity, proving that sustainable and nutritious choices can be deliciously intertwined.

3. Zero-Waste Veggie Broths and Flavorful Soups: The traditional concept of broth-making has undergone a sustainable makeover with the advent of zero-waste veggie broths. Collecting and freezing vegetable pulp over time transforms kitchen scraps into a rich and flavorful base for soups, stews, and risottos. This innovation not only maximizes the nutritional value of vegetables but also aligns with a zero-waste ethos. The resulting broths contribute depth and complexity to a variety of dishes, demonstrating that sustainable practices in the kitchen can lead to both culinary and environmental rewards.

4. Pioneering Plant-Based Patties and Fritters: In the realm of plant-based cuisine, sustainable and nutrient-rich culinary innovations extend to the creation of veggie patties and fritters. By combining leftover juicer pulp with grains, legumes, and aromatic spices, chefs are crafting savory and satisfying alternatives that challenge traditional notions of meat-centric dishes. These pioneering plant-based creations not only cater to a growing demand for sustainable protein sources but also celebrate the versatility of vegetable pulp in elevating the gastronomic experience. From veggie-packed patties to crispy fritters, these innovations showcase that sustainability and culinary delight can coexist on the same plate.

In the gastronomic landscape of sustainable and nutrient-rich culinary innovations, chefs and home cooks alike are pioneering a revolution that redefines the way we approach food. From repurposing juicer pulp to transforming breakfast rituals, creating zero-waste broths, and crafting plant-based patties, these culinary endeavors not only contribute to a more sustainable and mindful approach to cooking but also introduce a kaleidoscope of flavors and textures that tantalize the taste buds while nourishing the body. This gastronomic revolution proves that sustainable choices in the kitchen can be a delectable celebration of creativity and conscious living.

Chapter 8: Tips for Juicing on a Budget

Affordable and Accessible Nutrient-Rich Ingredients

Juicing on a budget doesn't mean compromising on nutrition or flavor. With strategic planning and a focus on affordable yet nutrient-dense ingredients, you can embrace the health benefits of juicing without breaking the bank.

1. Seasonal and Local Produce: Opt for seasonal and local fruits and vegetables to take advantage of lower prices and optimal freshness. Seasonal produce is often more abundant, making it more affordable, and local options can be found at farmers' markets or discount grocers. Incorporating what's in season not only supports your budget but also introduces variety into your juices based on what nature offers throughout the year.

2. Root Vegetables and Greens: Root vegetables like carrots, beets, and sweet potatoes are not only budget-friendly but also nutrient-dense, providing essential vitamins and minerals. Leafy greens, such as kale and spinach, are another affordable option that adds a nutritional punch to your juices. These ingredients are versatile, lending both sweetness and earthiness to your concoctions.

3. Buy in Bulk and Freeze: Purchase fruits and vegetables in bulk, especially when they are on sale or in-season. Freeze excess produce to prevent waste and ensure a steady supply of ingredients for your juices. Buying in bulk is often more cost-effective, and freezing allows you to stock up on items when prices are low, extending the lifespan of your budget-friendly juicing ingredients.

4. Incorporate Inexpensive Base Ingredients: Utilize cost-effective base ingredients to add volume and nutrients to your juices. Ingredients like apples, oranges, and cucumbers are not only affordable but also serve as excellent bases that complement a variety of other fruits and vegetables. These staples can be the backbone of your juice blends while allowing you to experiment with smaller amounts of pricier or more exotic ingredients.

5. Explore Frozen Fruits and Vegetables: Don't underestimate the value of frozen produce. Frozen fruits and vegetables can be more economical than fresh, and they offer the convenience of longer shelf life. Use frozen berries, mango chunks, or mixed vegetables to diversify your juice options without compromising on taste or nutritional content.

6. DIY Nut Milk and Seed Blends: Instead of buying expensive store-bought nut milks or seed blends, consider making your own at home. Purchase nuts, seeds, or grains in bulk and experiment with different combinations to create affordable and nutritious alternatives. Homemade nut and seed milks can add creaminess and flavor to your juices without the premium price tag.

7. Embrace Citrus for Flavor: Citrus fruits, such as oranges and lemons, are not only budget-friendly but also pack a flavorful punch. A little citrus zest or juice can enhance the taste of your juices without the need for additional sweeteners or expensive ingredients. Citrus fruits are often available year-round at reasonable prices.

8. *Mix High and Low-Cost Ingredients:* Strike a balance between high and low-cost ingredients to create budget-friendly yet nutritionally dense juice blends. Incorporate a small amount of pricier items, such as berries or tropical fruits, with more affordable staples like apples or carrots. This way, you can enjoy the flavors and benefits of various ingredients without overspending.

9. *Shop Sales and Discounts:* Keep an eye on sales, discounts, and promotions at your local grocery store. Many supermarkets offer weekly specials or discounts on bulk purchases. Planning your juicing ingredients around these promotions can significantly reduce your overall expenditure while still allowing for a diverse range of ingredients.

10. *Explore Ethnic or Discount Grocery Stores:* Consider exploring ethnic or discount grocery stores in your area. These establishments often provide a wide variety of fresh produce at lower prices compared to larger supermarkets. You may discover unique and cost-effective ingredients that can add diversity to your juicing routine.

By incorporating these budget-friendly tips into your juicing routine, you can savor the health benefits of nutrient-rich juices without straining your finances. With careful planning, a bit of creativity, and a focus on accessible ingredients, you'll find that juicing on a budget is not only feasible but also a delicious and rewarding endeavor.

Budget-Friendly Juicing Equipment and Tools

1. Entry-Level Juicers: When on a budget, opt for entry-level juicers that provide efficiency without compromising quality. Centrifugal juicers are often more affordable and readily available, offering a cost-effective solution for extracting juice from a variety of fruits and vegetables. These machines are user-friendly, easy to clean, and a great starting point for those embarking on their juicing journey without a hefty investment.

2. Manual Juicers and Citrus Presses: Consider manual juicers or citrus presses as economical alternatives, particularly if you primarily juice citrus fruits. These handheld devices are simple, easy to use, and require no electricity. Manual juicers, such as citrus reamers or handheld presses, efficiently extract juice from oranges, lemons, and limes without the need for a larger and more expensive electric juicer.

3. Blender or Food Processor: For those on an extremely tight budget, a blender or food processor can serve as a versatile substitute for a dedicated juicer. While the resulting concoction may retain more fiber than juice extracted from a traditional juicer, blending fruits and vegetables can still yield nutrient-rich and flavorful smoothies. This budget-friendly option allows you to embrace the benefits of homemade juices without the need for specialized equipment.

4. Thrifty Cutting Tools: Invest in budget-friendly cutting tools to prepare your fruits and vegetables before juicing. A reliable chef's knife, a sturdy cutting board, and a citrus zester are essential tools that can be acquired at reasonable prices. Efficiently chopping and preparing your produce ensures a smooth juicing process and contributes to the overall affordability of your juicing routine.

5. Glass Jars or Containers: When it comes to storing your freshly squeezed juices, opt for budget-friendly glass jars or containers. These reusable options are not only cost-effective but also eco-friendly, reducing the need for disposable containers. Glass jars with tight-fitting lids help preserve the freshness of your juices while being easy to clean and maintain.

6. Mesh Strainers or Cheesecloth: Strain your juices without the need for a specialized juice strainer by using budget-friendly mesh strainers or cheesecloth. These tools effectively separate the liquid from pulp, allowing you to achieve a smoother juice consistency without investing in additional and more expensive equipment. Mesh strainers and cheesecloth are readily available at affordable prices and can be used in various culinary applications.

7. Thrift Store Finds: Explore thrift stores or second-hand shops for potential budget-friendly juicing equipment. You may find gently used juicers, blenders, or cutting tools at a fraction of the cost. While ensuring that the equipment is in good condition, thrift store finds can be an excellent way to acquire essential juicing tools without breaking the bank.

Navigating a budget-friendly approach to juicing involves selecting accessible and affordable equipment that aligns with your financial constraints. Whether opting for entry-level juicers, manual presses, or improvising with basic kitchen tools, the key is to find options that cater to your juicing needs without compromising on the quality and nutritional value of your homemade concoctions.

Chapter 9: Juicing Safety and Precautions

Ensuring Hygiene in the Juicing Process

1. Wash Produce Thoroughly: Begin the hygiene process by washing all fruits and vegetables thoroughly before juicing. Use a produce brush for items with thicker skin, and consider using a mixture of water and vinegar to help remove pesticides and contaminants. This initial step ensures that the ingredients entering your juicer are free from dirt, bacteria, and surface residues.

2. Clean and Sanitize Equipment: Regularly clean and sanitize all juicing equipment, including the juicer, cutting boards, knives, and any other tools used in the process. Follow the manufacturer's instructions for disassembling and cleaning your juicer, paying extra attention to areas prone to pulp buildup. A mixture of warm water and mild dish soap or a vinegar solution can effectively remove any lingering residues and maintain a sanitary juicing environment.

3. Personal Hygiene: Prioritize personal hygiene to prevent the transfer of contaminants during the juicing process. Wash your hands thoroughly with soap and water before handling any ingredients or equipment. Consider using disposable gloves for an added layer of protection, especially if you have any cuts or abrasions on your hands.

4. Use Clean Cutting Surfaces: Ensure that all cutting surfaces, including cutting boards and countertops, are clean and sanitized before beginning the juicing process. Separate cutting boards for fruits and vegetables can prevent cross-contamination, and regularly disinfecting surfaces with a food-safe sanitizer or a mixture of water and white vinegar helps maintain a hygienic workspace.

5. Store Ingredients Properly: Store fruits and vegetables in a clean and refrigerated environment before juicing. Proper storage prevents the growth of harmful bacteria and ensures the freshness of your ingredients. Avoid using any produce that shows signs of spoilage or mold, as this can compromise the safety and quality of your juices.

6. Check and Clean Sieves and Strainers: Regularly inspect and clean sieves, strainers, and other juice-extracting components of your juicer. Pulp buildup in these areas can harbor bacteria and affect the cleanliness of your juices. Disassemble these parts according to the manufacturer's instructions, and clean them thoroughly after each juicing session.

7. Sanitize Glass Jars or Containers: If you plan to store your juices for later consumption, ensure that the glass jars or containers used for storage are properly sanitized. Run them through a dishwasher or hand wash with hot water and soap before filling them with freshly squeezed juice. This step prevents the growth of bacteria and maintains the hygiene of your stored juices.

8. Regular Appliance Maintenance: Follow a routine maintenance schedule for your juicing appliances. Regularly check for wear and tear, and replace any worn or damaged parts promptly. This proactive approach not only ensures the longevity of your equipment but also contributes to a cleaner and safer juicing process.

9. Hygienic Water Sources: If water is an ingredient in your juice or used to clean equipment, ensure that it comes from a safe and hygienic source. If using tap water, consider filtering it to remove impurities. Hygienic water minimizes the risk of introducing contaminants into your juices during the preparation and cleaning stages.

10. Dispose of Pulp and Waste Properly: Dispose of juicing waste, such as pulp and leftover produce, in a hygienic manner. Use designated compost bins or disposal bags to prevent cross-contamination and maintain a clean workspace. Regularly empty and clean the waste receptacles to prevent the buildup of odors and potential hygiene issues.

By incorporating these essential hygiene practices into your juicing routine, you not only ensure the safety of your homemade juices but also create a clean and sanitary environment in which to enjoy the nutritional benefits of fresh and wholesome ingredients.

Potential Interactions with Medications and Consulting Healthcare Professionals

Understanding Individual Health Profiles: Before incorporating juicing into your routine, it's crucial to recognize that certain fruits, vegetables, and herbs may interact with medications. Individual health profiles vary, and factors such as age, medical history, and specific medications can influence how the body processes substances. Engage in open communication with your healthcare provider about your intention to start juicing, providing them with a comprehensive overview of your medical history and the medications you are currently taking.

Identifying Medication-Juice Interactions: Certain compounds in fruits and vegetables, such as furanocoumarins in grapefruit, can interfere with drug metabolism. Grapefruit juice, in particular, is known to interact with a wide range of medications by inhibiting enzymes responsible for breaking down drugs in the liver. Other substances like leafy greens, high in vitamin K, can impact blood clotting and may interact with anticoagulant medications. It's essential to identify potential interactions to ensure the safe consumption of both medications and freshly squeezed juices.

Consulting Healthcare Professionals: Prioritize consultation with healthcare professionals before embarking on a significant dietary change, especially if you are managing chronic conditions or taking medications. Your healthcare provider can offer personalized guidance based on your specific health needs and prescribe adjustments to medication schedules or dosages if necessary. This proactive approach helps mitigate potential risks and ensures that juicing aligns with your overall healthcare plan.

Monitoring Blood Sugar Levels: For individuals with diabetes or those taking medications that affect blood sugar levels, closely monitor glucose levels when introducing freshly squeezed juices. Some fruits, despite their nutritional benefits, can cause spikes in blood sugar levels. Collaborate with healthcare professionals to establish a juicing plan that aligns with diabetes management goals, potentially incorporating low-glycemic fruits and vegetables.

Adapting to Individual Health Conditions: Individuals with kidney-related issues should be mindful of certain minerals in fruits and vegetables, as excessive intake may impact kidney function. Healthcare professionals can provide tailored advice to accommodate dietary restrictions or adjustments necessary for managing kidney health.

Balancing Nutrient Intake and Medications: Strive for a balance between nutrient-rich juices and the medications you are prescribed. Certain medications may require specific dietary considerations, such as taking them with or without food. Collaborate with healthcare providers to create a juicing plan that complements your medication regimen without compromising effectiveness.

Regular Medication Reviews: Engage in regular medication reviews with your healthcare team. As your health evolves, adjustments to medications or their interactions with freshly squeezed juices may be necessary. Periodic assessments ensure that your treatment plan aligns with your health goals and accommodates any dietary modifications.

In summary, while juicing offers numerous health benefits, it's crucial to approach dietary changes with caution, especially when managing chronic conditions or taking medications. Consulting healthcare professionals serves as a fundamental step in creating a safe and effective juicing plan tailored to individual health needs. Open communication, regular check-ins, and proactive adjustments contribute to a holistic approach that integrates juicing into a comprehensive healthcare strategy.

Conclusion

Recap of Key Principles and Takeaways

In summary, here are the key principles and takeaways when considering juicing, especially in the context of potential interactions with medications and overall health:

1. **Individualized Approach:**

   - Health profiles vary, and individual factors such as age, medical history, and medications influence how the body responds to dietary changes.

   - Adopt a personalized approach by consulting healthcare professionals before integrating juicing into your routine.

2. **Medication-Juice Interactions:**

   - Certain compounds in fruits and vegetables can interact with medications, potentially affecting drug metabolism.

   - Identify potential interactions, especially with substances like grapefruit juice, and collaborate with healthcare providers to mitigate risks.

3. **Open Communication with Healthcare Professionals:**

- Maintain open communication with healthcare providers about your intention to start juicing.

- Provide comprehensive information about your medical history, current medications, and any concerns or questions you may have.

4. **Blood Sugar Monitoring for Diabetes:**

- Individuals with diabetes or those on medications affecting blood sugar levels should monitor glucose levels when incorporating juices.

- Collaborate with healthcare professionals to create a juicing plan that aligns with diabetes management goals.

5. **Considerations for Kidney Health:**

- Individuals with kidney-related issues should be mindful of mineral intake from fruits and vegetables.

- Seek advice from healthcare professionals to adapt juicing plans based on kidney health considerations.

6. **Balancing Nutrient Intake:**

- Strive for a balance between nutrient-rich juices and prescribed medications.

- Collaborate with healthcare providers to ensure that juicing complements medication regimens without compromising effectiveness.

7. **Regular Medication Reviews:**

   - Engage in regular medication reviews with healthcare professionals to address any adjustments needed based on changing health conditions.

   - Periodic assessments ensure that your treatment plan aligns with health goals and accommodates any dietary modifications.

8. **Hygiene in the Juicing Process:**

   - Practice thorough hygiene by washing produce, cleaning and sanitizing equipment, and maintaining personal cleanliness.

   - Follow proper food safety measures to ensure the cleanliness and safety of freshly squeezed juices.

9. **Affordable Juicing Practices:**

   - Explore budget-friendly juicing equipment and tools, considering entry-level juicers, manual options, and DIY alternatives.

   - Utilize cost-effective ingredients, such as seasonal and local produce, to make juicing more affordable.

10. **Sustainable Juicing Habits:**

    - Embrace sustainability in juicing by repurposing leftover pulp and exploring creative recipes.

- Practice mindful waste disposal and consider thrifty options for equipment to reduce environmental impact.

By incorporating these principles into your juicing journey, you can navigate potential challenges, prioritize health and safety, and enjoy the nutritional benefits of freshly squeezed juices in a sustainable and personalized manner. Always consult with healthcare professionals for tailored advice and guidance.

Embracing a Healthier Future through Juicing

In the pursuit of a healthier future, juicing emerges as a vibrant and transformative avenue towards holistic well-being. Beyond the refreshing taste of freshly squeezed juices, this practice embodies a commitment to nourishing the body with an abundance of vitamins, minerals, and antioxidants derived from nature's bounty. The essence lies not only in the vibrant hues of fruits and vegetables but in the profound impact on overall health. Embracing juicing means embracing a lifestyle that prioritizes personalized nutrition, mindful dietary choices, and a conscious connection to the earth's offerings. It is a journey where each sip becomes a testament to the body's resilience and its capacity for rejuvenation. As we blend and extract the vibrant life force from fruits and vegetables, we embark on a path that nurtures not only physical vitality but also a deeper sense of well-being. Through this ritual of self-care, we pave the way for a healthier, more vibrant future, where every glass of juice becomes a celebration of the body's innate ability to thrive and flourish.